Gut Health and Probiotics

'Happiness starts with
a happy gut!

Leny

Gut Health and Probiotics

The Science Behind the Hype

Jenny Tschiesche

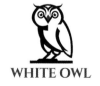

WHITE OWL

First published in Great Britain in 2018 by
PEN & SWORD WHITE OWL
An imprint of
Pen & Sword Books Ltd
Yorkshire - Philadelphia

ISBN 978 1 52672 045 0

A CIP catalogue record for this book is available from the British Library

Typeset in Times New Roman 10.5/13 by
Aura Technology and Software Services, India
Printed and bound in India by Replika Press Pvt. Ltd.

Pen & Sword Books Ltd incorporates the Imprints of Aviation, Atlas,
Family History, Fiction, Maritime, Military, Discovery, Politics, History,
Archaeology, Select, Wharncliffe Local History, Wharncliffe True Crime,
Military Classics, Wharncliffe Transport, Leo Cooper, The Praetorian Press,
Remember When, Seaforth Publishing and Frontline Publishing.

For a complete list of Pen & Sword titles please contact

PEN & SWORD BOOKS LTD
47 Church Street, Barnsley, South Yorkshire, S70 2AS, England
E-mail: enquiries@pen-and-sword.co.uk
Website: www.pen-and-sword.co.uk

Or

PEN AND SWORD BOOKS
1950 Lawrence Rd, Havertown, PA 19083, USA
E-mail: Uspen-and-sword@casematepublishers.com
Website: www.penandswordbooks.com

Contents

Biography:

Jenny Tschiesche is one of the UK's leading nutrition experts and the founder of www.lunchboxdoctor.com, (a popular resource for parents and teachers who want to learn more about good health and nutrition.) She creates delicious recipes and health campaigns for big companies, including BBC Sport, Sport England, Cancer Research UK and The Realbuzz Group. Jenny regularly contributes to radio and television shows, such as *Good Morning Britain* and to newspapers and magazines like *The Guardian, The Daily Mail, Prima* and *Top Santé*. In addition to this new book on Gut Health and Probiotics, Jenny has created two recipe books. Both are being published in 2018. The first book is called SHEET PAN COOKING 101 recipes for simple and nutritious meals straight from the oven.

Brief Introduction:

A simplified explanation of probiotics, and what they can do for the human body, is long overdue. Despite the fact that people are now used to the term, they seem unsure whether probiotics occur naturally in a healthy human gut or 'biome', something that is added to yogurt or simply some sort of medicine. This book will take readers on a quest to understand what both **probiotics** and **prebiotics** can do for their long-term gut health and the effects this might have on just about every part of their bodies. Along the way, readers will discover how useful probiotics can be in both preventing and curing specific ailments. There's also the chance to understand more about where you can find both prebiotics and probiotics and how they have been used traditionally for centuries.

Foreword
by Cyndi O'Meara- Australia's Premier Nutritionist, author, speaker, educator and documentary maker

Nutrigenomics, epigenetics, microbiome, microbiota, GUT, zonulin, lactobacillus, bifidus, autoimmunity, antibiotic resistant, glyphosate, dysbiosis, leaky gut are words becoming common terms in nutrition and for people seeking health.

I've been a nutritionist for over three decades, I graduated with a Bachelor of Science majoring in Nutrition from Deakin University, I studied anthropology and human anatomy at other universities and the only word in the above list that was uttered in my 6 years of science was GUT. Back then it was called the GIT.

We have a whole new language in nutrition and a plethora of information that is growing exponentially every year about the GUT, and there is a very good reason.

Over the past two decades GUT issues are on the rise, many people have been given diagnosis, suffering with bloating, constipation, diarrhea, coeliac disease, fructose malabsorption, leaky gut, intestinal permeability, Crohns disease, ulcerative colitis, SIBO (small intestinal bacteria overgrowth), fat malabsorption, indigestion and cancers of the alimentary canal. This is by no means a full list, but common words we now hear.

There has also been a steady rise in systemic diseases including heart disease, diabetes, cancer and autoimmunity. Autoimmunity is a blanket term including one hundred plus diseases most notably, multiple sclerosis, type 1 diabetes, lupus, hashimotos, graves, addisons, parkinsons and rheumatoid arthritis.

Hippocrates is the father of medicine, medical doctors take the Hippocratic oath on graduation. We know the words "first do no harm". Hippocrates also said "all disease begins in the GUT". These words were said over 2000 years ago but none are truer than what we know today.

Modern medicine has taken only part of what this great man had to say and has forgotten that the food we eat and GUT health are vital for health.

Until recently most patients went to their doctor, described their symptoms, were diagnosed with a condition or disease, and then treated with a medication and told that diet had nothing to do with their disease or symptoms. And just quietly I still hear that this is going on.

Let's just think about the first part of this statement for a minute. It's like saying the red light on the dash board of your motor vehicle, which indicates a problem, just needs a piece of cardboard over it to hide the indicator. It's like putting your head in the sand and not acknowledging that a symptom is an indicator to the body that something is wrong, and then dulling the symptom with a medication, let's explore the cause of the problem.

The second part of the statement is like saying that the petrol you put into a diesel car will not affect its performance. Well that's just plain silly! Of course it will. The food you put in your body affects every cell and it's biochemistry, thus affecting every system and organ. Not only do we know that the food we eat can help us with energy and building blocks for the body but we now know that every food we consume affects our DNA. Food communicates with our DNA, our blueprint for life. It can turn on or off the messages that DNA gives the body in order to be healthy or sick, this is the wonderful new science of nutrigenomics.

A good friend of mine is a gastroenterologist and recently I asked him about his university days and what he was taught about food and the GUT. He told me he was taught to diagnose and treat diseases of the GUT, he was not given any information about how food affected the GUT and thus the health of an individual.

But times are changing; research is showing that the GUT has everything to do with not only physical health but also mental health.

It's all very well and good to understand the anatomy and physiology of the GUT but what is becoming a burgeoning science, is the ecology of the GUT.

The GUT has a group of residents, including; bacteria, viruses, parasites, fungi and yeasts. These microbes are called the microbiota, their genetic makeup is ten times greater than the genetic makeup of the human they reside within. These bugs live symbiotically with us, helping us digest, fight off infection, make vitamins, amino acids, fats and much more. We cannot live without our microbiota. The health of your microbiota is important for your health.

Our current lifestyle, of food produced with chemicals, chemicals in the environment and in our home, the overuse of antibiotics, the consumption of food like substances, refined and packaged foods, lack of sleep and exercise, not enough sunlight, all contribute to a microbiota that falls into dysbiosis (sick). As the GUT and the microbiota get sick so do we.

Jenny Tschiesche has mastered the knowledge of the GUT, it's ecology and it's affect on human health. This wonderful book is not only an important resource for the lay person, but should be compulsory reading for every health professional whether graduated or still at university. The information is succinct many with citations. I will be recommending this book to all my students at the Functional Nutrition Academy.

Not only does Jenny impress upon us how the GUT and microbiome is being eroded and why we are seeing an increase in GUT issues, but she also gives solid advice on how we can improve the integrity of the GUT and microbiota.

Thomas A Edison said "The doctor of the future will give no medication, but will interest his patients in the care of the human frame, diet and in the cause and prevention of disease" This future has come, and this book will be a valuable resource to lead the way.

Thank you Jenny for putting the hard work in, all the research and simply explaining this massive, important subject.

Cyndi O'Meara
BSc Nutritionist
Founder of Changing Habits and Functional Nutritional Academy
Producer and Director of the documentary "What's With Wheat"
Author of Changing Habits Changing Lives
Australia's Leading Nutritionist

Chapter 1

Gut Health and the Modern Way of Living

Think of all those well-known phrases with gut at the core – 'a gut reaction', 'gut decision', 'spill your guts'. Gut is a well-used word and yet do we ever stop to think about what we are really referring to? The technical definition, if you choose to look it up on one of the world's most well-known search engines is 'the alimentary canal, especially between the pylorus and the anus, or some portion of it.' Even that definition seems rather ambiguous – further proof that this book needed to be written in the first place. What is our gut? What do we mean when we talk about 'good gut health'? Where do probiotics fit into all of this?

Ask most people what 'probiotics' are and they might refer to the 'tummy-friendly bacteria' in the small yogurt drinks they've seen advertised. Some might talk about natural yogurt providing good bacteria and others might refer to probiotic supplements that can be taken when you have an upset stomach – this idea of course being based on a commonly held belief that there's a 'pill for an ill'. In fact, if your health-related news antennae are particularly active, then you may have picked up on the fact that some nutritional experts are referring to probiotics as the 'health foods of the year'. As a whole range of ready-made probiotic foods hit the market from kefir to kombucha and recipe books on the subject of fermented foods gain popularity, it really is time to discover what probiotics actually are.

Perhaps one reason for such confusion is that we are skewed towards thinking of ill health as something that can be fixed by medication rather than focussing on prevention of illness. The prevention of ill health is behind many of the food preparation practices from more traditional cultures, which tend to produce naturally probiotic-rich foods. Names like Lactobacillus acidophilus, Lactobacillus brevis or Lactobacillus casei might not have be familiar to the people making kefir on a regular basis in the past they just knew it did them good. More traditional cultures where

1

probiotic-rich (fermented) foods are commonplace view these foods not only as necessary but also as preventative.

According to the World Health Organisation 'health is a state of complete physical, mental and social wellbeing, and not merely the absence of disease or infirmity.' But our more modern food processing techniques don't really lend themselves to this ethos.

Our lifestyles today include the consumption of large amounts of sugar-loaded, additive-filled, overly-processed foods, and high levels of the wrong kinds of fats such as trans fats (found in cheap baked goods) and oxidised fats created by heating or frying food in vegetable oils. Yet it wasn't so long ago that we were enjoying slow-cooked stews and casseroles, and eating nose-to-tail – having the whole animal including the liver, tongue, kidney and heart, drinking live yogurt which hadn't had the 'good bacteria' added in because the natural methods of production had put it there in the first place, and consuming sourdough bread that took five days to develop even the 'starter' that was used in place of modern, fast-acting yeast.

When you think that much of what we consume today, such as breakfast cereals, fizzy drinks, low-fat spread, artificial sweeteners, excess alcohol, and even infant formula was unknown to our bodies just a hundred years ago it makes sense that the introduction of these new compounds might explain the increase in food intolerance and allergies. Our gut simply can't cope.

Add to that the ubiquitous prescription of antibiotics, the long-term use of birth control pills, and the use of over the counter pain relievers and possibly other medication, the gut (or 'microbiome' as we should refer to it) is left damaged and that exposes us to more infections and makes us vulnerable to other health issues too.

It doesn't stop with food and medication either. Our gut bacteria vary depending on age, gender, geography, hygiene, stress, birthing method (C-section or vaginal delivery) and our first foods (breast milk or formula). They can all determine what bacteria colonise our gut.

An imbalance of gut bacteria has been related to a wide variety of ailments that may seem entirely unrelated to the gut. As we will see over the course of this book, it can lead to mental health problems, autism, high cholesterol, achy joints and many autoimmune conditions to name a few.

This concept of gut imbalance has been so widely studied by scientists that it has its own name. It is called 'dysbiosis', a word first coined by scientist Dr Eli Metchnikoff in the early 1920s. It is derived from two words 'symbiosis' meaning living together in mutual harmony and 'dis' which means not. Yet we cannot talk about the health issues related to dysbiosis without referring briefly to the connection between an imbalance of gut bacteria and a condition called Leaky Gut Syndrome.

Leaky Gut Syndrome

This is a condition which is not always recognised by mainstream medical professionals. However, the evidence of its existence and its link to a number of illnesses is mounting rapidly. Leaky gut occurs when the gut becomes overloaded by stress, toxins, drugs, pathogenic bacteria and poor food choices. When this combines with a low number of beneficial gut bugs and a lack of diversity then gaps can form between the cells lining the gut, called epithelial cells.

A leaky gut is not a loyal gut. It might shut the gates to beneficial nutrients while welcoming dangerous bacteria inside. Gaps in the periphery of the gut also let in viruses which might otherwise be dealt with by the gut bacteria. Now that these bacteria and viruses can access the body via the bloodstream they pose a far bigger threat to health. This movement across the lining of the gut into the bloodstream is called 'bacterial translocation' or BT for short.

Leaky Gut Progression

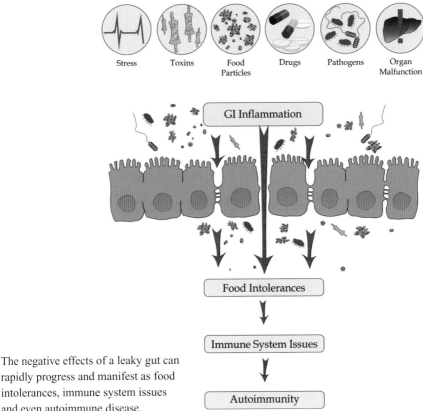

| Stress | Toxins | Food Particles | Drugs | Pathogens | Organ Malfunction |

GI Inflammation

Food Intolerances

Immune System Issues

Autoimmunity

The negative effects of a leaky gut can rapidly progress and manifest as food intolerances, immune system issues and even autoimmune disease.

What gut bacteria do for you?

We are discovering so much more about the role of gut health in our overall health thanks to scientists now focusing specifically on this area. We've realised that our gut bacteria are instrumental for some seriously life-sustaining functions. Some of the most important functions identified so far relate to:

- Immune system function
- Controlling inflammation
- Improving the rate of detoxification
- Improving mood by playing a role in the production of our 'happy hormone' serotonin
- Making vitamins, including B vitamins like folate, biotin and B12 as well as vitamin K2
- Preventing the development or worsening of leaky gut
- Improving nutrient absorption, especially of iron, zinc and magnesium

You are what you eat

Each human has a very individual health profile and balance of bacteria. However we are all very much the product of our environment, and specifically our dietary choices, when it comes to bacterial balance. You may have heard of the phrase, 'You are what you eat'. This adage seems more apt now than ever. Study after study has revealed a clear link between dietary choices and gut bacteria. Our food choices have a profound effect on the diversity of our gut microbes – and more diversity means a healthier microbiome.

One 2015 study[1] showed that Americans who ate diets formed predominantly of processed fast foods had significantly limited bacterial diversity in their guts when compared to South Africans whose diets were higher in fibre. The fascinating part of this particular study was that within two weeks of switching diets the situation started to improve for those who normally ate a fast food diet and were now eating more like the South African participants. Equally the markers for good gut health were lower in the South African participants who had switched to the American diet after the same two week period. The speed of positive change related to dietary changes is exciting as far as disease prevention is concerned and even as far as achieving optimal health. The speed of microbiome health recovery seems extraordinary but it is another reminder of just how adaptive and responsive the human body can be to positive health interventions.

What we cannot fail to identify is that the modern Western diet is very far away from the real food diet of our ancestors. When I say ancestors I am not talking about those members of our families who lived millions of years ago.

I am instead referring to those who may simply have lived a hundred years ago. If they were to walk into a modern supermarket or a fast food restaurant of today would they even recognise what we are eating as food? Even if they did, they may question where it has come from and what we have done to it. As a society, we are very far removed from the source of our food. Most of us have no idea where our meat is farmed or our vegetables picked. Furthermore we have no idea about the processing that goes on before a particular food in its packaging makes it onto the shelves of our favoured supermarket.

A case in point is cured meat. Curing would have been a very familiar process to our ancestors a century ago. They would probably have cured meat, fish and vegetables themselves. However as demand increased for cured meats and sausages so the process moved out of the home and into the factories. The use of nitrates in this environment became commonplace but was unregulated until scientists realised that the nitrosamines, that form when nitrites are present in high concentrations and the product is cooked at high temperatures, could be cancerous. In fact, according to World Cancer Research Fund analysis those who eat the most processed meats have around a 17% higher risk of developing bowel cancer than those who eat the least processed meats. To give you an idea of the potential impact of nitrosamines on health of a population, since the European Union stipulated that cured products should contain no more than100mg of nitrate salts per 1kg of meat, the rates of stomach cancer in Europe have fallen considerably. Our modern tastes are beyond our knowledge of what's healthy and actually what's doing us harm.

You are a product of your environment

It appears that where we live in the world and what we may be exposed to in our environment can play a part in the gut bacteria we play host to. For example in a *New Scientist*[2] article regarding the possibility that gut health and Parkinson's disease may be closer linked than we initially thought, it was noted that farmers exposed to certain pesticides, and people who get their drinking water from wells – which might be contaminated with pesticides – are more likely to get Parkinson's. It was concluded that these chemicals can also damage nerves in the gut so the relationship between gut health and the development of Parkinson's may be initially triggered by environmental toxins. Many studies have shown that where populations have lived in a largely unchanged culture and environment for some time their gut bacteria appears to be both stable and healthy. However when industrial foods grown using chemicals, processed in factories and created for mass consumption came along and when medications such as pain relievers and antibiotics entered the frame changed and the gut bacteria of the population changes too.

Mood and gut health

Serotonin is well known as a neurotransmitter. However, what is less well known is that an estimated ninety per cent of the body's serotonin is produced in the digestive tract. Taking this into consideration, when you think of people who have poor digestion they often have low mood problems too. It is hardly a surprise. In fact, probiotics have been shown to improve anxiety in animal-based studies[3]. Further human studies have revealed that probiotics can have a direct effect on brain chemistry, impacting feelings of anxiety or depression. A 2013 study[4] even showed a relationship between prebiotic supplements and anxiety in so far as the prebiotics appeared to alter the way that people processed emotional information. The relationship between probiotics and prebiotics is discussed later on in this book but it seems that both can have a positive effect on mind symptoms.

How our understanding of gut bacteria and disease is advancing

Our understanding of what other diseases may be linked to gut health is advancing at a pace. The possible relationship between Parkinson's and the gut was first discovered about ten years before the *New Scientist* [5] article. This was when autopsies revealed the very substance associated with Parkinson's - clumps of synuclein that were normally found within the brain, were discovered in the nerves of the gut. Of course, it would be hard to find out if these clumps of fibres travel from the gut to the brain in human beings but tests have been carried out on mice that show this to be the case. The mice in one particular study became less agile, something that happens to humans with Parkinson's disease. Scientists made a further correlation between Parkinson's sufferers and gut problems in the period leading up to diagnosis. People diagnosed with Parkinson's often report digestive issues, most commonly constipation, in the ten years leading up to the first tremors. Our knowledge[6] relating to probiotics shows that they may be able to positively influence the gut bacteria of potential Parkinson's sufferers and could change the outcomes of this illness.

Another disease that has recently been linked to changes in the microbiome is type 1 diabetes. In a 2016 study[7], researchers followed children who were genetically predisposed to the condition. They found that onset for those who developed the disease was preceded by a drop in microbial diversity. Scientist Alexandra Paun[8], in her 2016 paper, goes as far as to suggest that the association between changes in gut microbiota and both diabetes type 1 and type 2 is so strong that microbe-derived medication could potentially be used for prevention and/or treatment of both conditions in the future. Furthermore, a group of researchers from the US Argonne National Laboratory discovered that gut bacteria (in particular bacterial enzymes) could affect the process of breaking down sugars into glucose. This discovery could have implications for the treatment of diabetes.

> *'Much of the medicine prescribed today focuses on human, rather than bacterial, cells. We target human enzymes with drugs, but we don't often target bacterial enzymes. If someone has diabetes, doctors prescribe drugs to control their production of glucose. We might want to consider whether bacterial enzymes that produce glucose should also be targeted.'* Andzej Joachimiak, Argonne National Laboratory

In summary, our modern lifestyles and dietary choices are having a major impact on our overall health. The places we choose to live, the jobs we do, the stress we put our bodies under, the foods we eat all play a part in the development of our gut bacteria over time and this can in turn affect our future health in ways we probably never thought possible. We must open our minds to the possibility that 'poor gut health' doesn't mean a bit of tummy ache or the odd bout of diarrhoea or constipation. Nor does it mean a little indigestion or acid reflux when we have consumed too many spicy meals or alcohol. Gut problems really do extend way beyond the gut. As we go through this book, we shall go on a journey to understand exactly how important the bacteria in our gut really are to our overall health and wellbeing. We will look at what happens when we have too few 'good' and too many 'bad' bacteria present and how we might be able to use our knowledge to address imbalances that may be the cause of major disease. To do this properly, we shall have to rely on the hard evidence available, the science behind the myths, and not our "gut feeling".

Chapter 2

A Journey through the Digestive System

In order to appreciate the role of probiotics and prebiotics in gut health, it is important to understand how the digestive system works. It might help to think of the upper gut as an almost sterile, digesting, carnivorous organ (like a dog's or a cat's), evolved to deal with meat and fat, whilst the lower gut (large bowel or colon) is full of bacteria and is a fermenting, vegetarian gut (like a horse or cow's), evolved to digest vegetables and fibre.

	Characteristics
Upper Gut	Few Bacteria - Almost Sterile
	Digesting
	Carnivorous
Lower Gut	Loads of Bacteria
	Fermenting
	Vegetarian

Components of the Digestive System

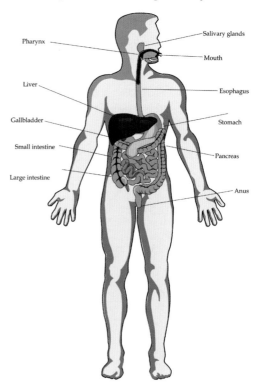

Your digestive system is essentially a tube that runs from your mouth to your anus. The tube runs through various different 'departments' and each has a role to play for optimal digestion to take place. If everything runs smoothly and the departments work effectively together then things go well. If not, then digestion will not be effective and ill health may well result.

The mouth

Digestion begins in the mouth. This is where the food first starts to get broken down. The processes involved in this first stage are grinding and chewing of the food by our teeth and enzymatic breakdown (our saliva contains enzymes that start to break the food down into smaller molecules so that our body can absorb the nutrients in the food efficiently). Saliva is sometimes produced even when we start to think about tasty food, but certainly when we smell it, see it and start to cook it. In fact, both cooking and eating slowly (or 'mindfully') can aid overall digestion. Yet, many of us don't cook and we certainly don't tend to eat slowly or mindfully either. Modern lunches tend to be a rushed affair. Often the same food will be eaten day in day out, in large gulps as we respond to urgent emails or check out social media updates. Breakfast is often on the run as few people have time to sit down and eat before they leave the house. And evening meals are frequently eaten in front of the television or as we're glued to devices. None of these eating environments are really suited to optimal digestion because, put simply, your body is focused on things other than digesting food.

> '*Fear less, hope more; eat less, chew more; whine less, breathe more; talk less, say more; hate less, love more; and all good things will be yours.*' Swedish Proverb

The stomach

After the initial breakdown of food in the mouth by the teeth and the saliva, the food travels down a stretchy pipe known as the oesophagus. Muscles in the wall of the oesophagus move food along in waves. At the end of this pipe, the food reaches the stomach. The stomach sits behind the ribs and is an extendible sack shaped like the letter J. When someone says, 'I've got stomach ache,' and move their hands towards their torso, it rarely comes to rest on their actual stomach. In fact, people often seem surprised when you point out just how high up the stomach actually is. Quite often, actual 'stomach ache' occurs further down the gastrointestinal tract.

The stomach stretches to accommodate larger quantities of food. Here the food gets tossed around like clothes in a washing machine, using the muscles of the stomach wall to spur this motion on. This process helps to break the food down even further. The stomach produces a powerful acid called hydrochloric acid and even more enzymes, called digestive enzymes. This combination of chemicals and physical churning breaks the food down into a sloppy mass which then moves to the small intestine.

If, however, your gut is not in perfect health you may not produce sufficient hydrochloric acid or digestive enzymes. This is a very common contributor to the symptoms associated with Irritable Bowel Syndrome, as both insufficiencies will result in sluggish digestion that means that food stays in the wrong place for too long. Furthermore, if you have not chewed your food sufficiently or have eaten under stressful conditions, gulping air with each mouthful and not allowing your body to produce sufficient stomach acid and enzymes to break down your food, problems can occur. When undigested food hangs around in the stomach for too long it starts to putrefy.

The small intestine

The name 'small' intestine implies that this part of the body plays a far less significant part in processing food than it actually does. But the small intestine is not small by most standards. In fact it is about six metres long. It also plays an important role in the absorption of nutrients from food. After all, this is the reason we need to eat in the first place. We need to absorb nutrients for our survival.

At this point, the pre-digested sloppy mass is given a name. It is called 'chyme', and at the same time, an important digestive chemical called bile is released by the gallbladder and more enzymes join in to help break down the chyme into smaller particles. It is from these smaller particles that we can absorb nutrients into our bloodstream.

The tube that is your small intestine is lined with finger-like projections called villi and on each villi, there are even smaller finger-like projections called micro villi. The reason for the existence of these finger-like projections is to increase the surface area of the intestine further. This means there is even more opportunity for the nutrients from the chyme to be absorbed.

Chyme moves through the small intestine at regular intervals throughout the day and the cells of the tube have to work hard, so hard that they get worn down easily. So the cells of the villi and microvilli get replaced regularly in a healthy digestive system. They are further helped and protected by a mucus that coats the villi and microvilli, protecting them and preventing the pathogenic bacteria and yeast that are travelling though the digestive system from being absorbed.

A poorly operating digestive system may have a low turnover of the cells forming the microvilli and villi, or may not be producing sufficient mucus for protection. Any one of these issues, and certainly a combination of more than one of them, will lead to poor absorption of nutrients from the food we eat. The degree to which this occurs determines just how sick we might become. As the nutrients make their way out of the small intestine via the villi and microvilli, the rest of the undigested food travels onwards to the large intestine.

The large intestine

The large intestine is also known as the colon. It is almost the end of the line for the food, which is now very much broken down and sloppy in consistency. Our large intestine is actually shorter than the small intestine but it is known as the 'large' intestine because it is very much wider. As you know, what is ultimately released from our bodies (in the form of stools) is not sloppy or certainly shouldn't be in a healthy body with an efficient digestive system. One of the roles that the large intestine plays is to absorb the excess water from the sloppy mass. This water can then be reused for other processes in the body. However, the large intestine also plays host to literally trillions of microbes. They interact with the food particles that still may not have been broken down. A process called bacterial fermentation converts the chyme into faeces and releases vitamins K, B1, B2, B6, B12, and biotin. Vitamin K is almost exclusively produced by the gut bacteria and is essential in the clotting of blood. Those whose diets are nutrient-poor may rely on these bacteria-derived vitamins for optimal health. However, antibiotics will easily wipe out the bacteria responsible for this fermentation process. Therefore both diet and supplementation should be reviewed post antibiotics in order to restore nutrient levels.

Although bacteria exist throughout the whole digestive system the majority reside here in the large intestine. The roles played by these bacteria are far wider than many of us ever realised in the past. Even as recently as ten years ago, the link between gut bacteria and obesity for example was little known, let alone recognised and researched. Now we know that the microbes of the large intestine are linked to feelings of satiety (being satisfied by the quantity of food consumed) and hunger. Gut microbes interact with the hormones ghrelin and leptin which in turn can communicate whether we are hungry or satisfied. Having a healthy balance of bacteria in the large intestine can allow for optimal calorie consumption. Of course, the inverse is also true – a poor balance of bacteria in this part of the gastrointestinal tract may slow down the rate at which calories are used by the body. Today we have an abundance of studies that show us that the role of large intestine microbes is broad in range and deep in terms of the effect on our overall health and wellbeing and yes, they can affect our body weight too.

The microbes in the large intestine play a role in fermenting indigestible fibres from predominantly vegetable sources. Remember this is the 'vegetarian' part of the digestive tract (more akin to the gut of a cow or horse). The product of this fermentation process is most often a substance called butyrate. Butyrate helps improve the concentration of mucus which lines the gut and protects the body from pathogens. A diet without vegetables would leave someone lacking in their ability to produce sufficient mucus to line the digestive tract. This would make them more vulnerable to poor digestion, ill health and importantly Leaky Gut Syndrome. The standout message here is that vegetables must be a part of a healthy, balanced diet in order to help balance gut bacteria.

How long does it take for food to be digested?
The action of food being processed and then moving on to the next part of the digestive tract is quite lengthy. On average, it might take up to two days from ingestion of food to excretion from the body as stools.

50% of stomach contents emptied	2.5 to 3 hours
Total emptying of the stomach	4 to 5 hours
50% emptying of the small intestine	2.5 to 3 hours
Transit through the colon	30 to 40 hours

Digestion
For optimal health, it's not just a question of what we eat but how well our body digests that food. Digestion is simply the process of breaking food and drink down into smaller particles so that they can be absorbed into the body. The process of digestion varies according to the food group being broken down (i.e. protein, carbohydrate, or fat). The products of digestion (amino acids, glucose, and fatty acids) are used by the body as building blocks for everything the body makes.

- Amino acids build proteins. Proteins are what the majority of the solids inside the body's cells are made up of. This includes muscles, collagen, hormones, neurotransmitters and immune system antibodies.
- Glucose is the sugar that the body uses to convert into cellular energy. About twenty-five per cent of the body's entire glucose production is used by the brain.
- Fatty acids and lipids can be broken down into glucose, but are also used to make cell membranes as well as nerve sheaths, steroid hormones and cholesterol. Fats have a very important part to play in our overall health and wellbeing, and in particular our immunity, because they help form the lipid bi-layer (a double layer of fatty acids) at our cell membranes. These membranes become selectively permeable. This means that they allow certain things into the cells while keeping other things out.

The rate at which digestion occurs and how efficient this process is depends on the balance of gut bacteria throughout the digestive tract. In short, it depends on the state of the 'microbiome'.

The Microbiome – a new term

This term was first coined by American scientist Joshua Lederberg in 2001. It is defined as 'the ecological community of commensal, symbiotic, and pathogenic microorganisms that literally 'share our body space'. It is now used to refer to both the bacteria and their associated genes. You may also hear the term microbiota which some scientists use to refer to only the microbes within the microbiome.

The microbiome is now of such importance that people talk about it being an organ in its own right. That seems fitting when you consider that researchers now calculate that more than 10,000 microbial species occupy the human ecosystem. Moreover, scientists calculate that the human genome carries some 22,000 protein-coding genes, whilst they believe that the human microbiome contributes some 8 million unique protein-coding genes or 360 times more bacterial genes than human genes. There is some research now emerging to suggest that these gut bacteria genes interact with

YOUR MICROBIOME

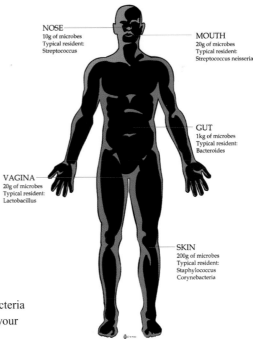

NOSE
10g of microbes
Typical resident:
Streptococcus

MOUTH
20g of microbes
Typical resident:
Streptococcus neisseria

GUT
1kg of microbes
Typical resident:
Bacteroides

VAGINA
20g of microbes
Typical resident:
Lactobacillus

SKIN
200g of microbes
Typical resident:
Staphylococcus
Corynebacteria

Microbiome refers not only to the bacteria in your gut but also on your skin, in your mouth, nose and vagina.

our human genes to switch them on or off. This is another way in which gut bacteria could play a key role in the existence or not of diseases in any one human being.

In summary, the digestive process starts as soon as we start to even think about food and each part of the digestive tract literally feeds the next so each department must be healthy and operating smoothly for optimal digestion. Poor digestion is linked to a multitude of factors, many within our direct control, including stress levels and eating when distracted and not relaxed. In order to make sure quality food is properly digested by your digestive system it is important first to make healthier food and drink choices. This means having a varied diet rich in good quality proteins and fats, rich in plant-based foods that can provide the fuel (or prebiotics) for probiotics to thrive. It is also important to eat in an environment free from work or other distractions, and to eat mindfully, allowing your digestive system to focus on the task in hand.

Chapter 3

Why do I have bugs in my body?

There are more bacteria in your intestinal tract than there are cells in your body. However astonishing this seems, facts about our microbiome are emerging at such a rate that we are starting to truly understand the importance of these living organisms and why they play such a significant part in our overall health and wellbeing.

Gut Bacteria Facts:
• There are 100 trillion bacteria living in our digestive tracts
• Gut bacteria are 10-50 times smaller than human cells
• The total weight of these bacteria is 4lbs – that's about the same weight as your liver
• 80% of the dry weight of your stool is composed of bacteria

Whilst we tend to hear mostly about two main gut bacteria (lactobacilli and bifidobacterium) there are many more different types. Scientists estimate that we have more than 10,000 microbial species. The possible permutations are so numerous as to make us all unique in terms of our own gut flora. That fact alone can make optimising gut bacteria a very personal crusade to wellness. What is becoming apparent is that there may be some correlation between groups of people who have similar (but not identical) gut bacteria profiles and the kinds of illnesses those groups are prone to. From a diagnostic perspective, this is an exciting area of development. We shall be discovering more about this in Chapter 5.

The main strains of bacteria:
1. Bacteroides
2. Bifidobacteria
3. Eubacterium
4. Fusobacteria

The main strains of bacteria:
5. Lactobacillus
6. Peptococcaceae
7. Ruminococcus
8. Streptococcus

These bacteria are not all located in the same part of the gastrointestinal tract. They tend to prefer different environments, depending on the nature of each strain. This is where you'll find the main strains within the digestive system.

Intestinal Microflora

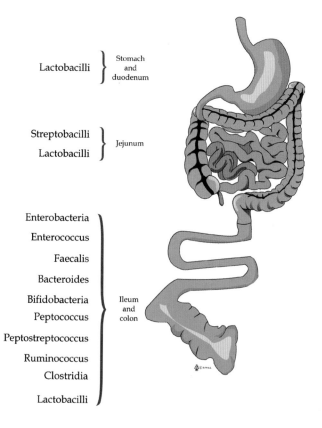

The number of bacteria naturally present throughout our digestive tract:

Mouth	Stomach	Small Intestine	Large Intestine
Billions	Few	Multiple Billions	Trillions and Trillions

Where do the bacteria come from?
Mother's diet
Whilst we are in our mother's womb we are fed pre-digested foods via the placenta. Scientists used to believe that babies were born with sterile guts and had no need for gut bacteria of their own. However recent research[9] suggests that we are already starting to develop a unique set of gut bacteria whilst in utero, from our mother's digestive system. These bacteria are affected by the mother's diet and lifestyle, and have been linked to an increased risk of the baby developing various types of health issues. This new research means that what a mother eats and her lifestyle choices are already starting to develop a baby's gut bacteria in the womb. These findings could have a great impact on the advice offered to newly pregnant women.

Birthing method
As a baby travels down the birth canal the process of gut bacteria colonisation, which started in the womb, progresses at a pace. This means that the mode of birth can make a difference to the type and quantity of gut bacteria because some babies are not born via the birth canal. Whilst infants born naturally have been shown to acquire vaginal lactobacilli from the mother those born via caesarean section (C-section) may acquire staphylococcus bacteria from the mother's skin flora. Furthermore, when researchers compared children who had been born vaginally with children who had been delivered by C-section they found the latter had less diverse flora, lower levels of Shigella bacteria and none of the bacteria known as Bacteroides.[10] Both Shigella and Bacteroides are organisms picked up from the mother and are considered first colonisers. To the best of our current knowledge, these bacteria are required to lay the foundation for further microbes that become part of a normal, healthy microbiome. Taking this into consideration it is fair to say that children born via C-section may be at a disadvantage when it comes to gut bacterial diversity. This may make them more susceptible to ill health as it is easier for pathogenic bacteria to colonise when there's less resistance from host bacteria.

Formula or breastfed and gut bacteria
Gut colonisation continues as a baby starts to feed. There are bacteria in both breast milk and formula milk. There are also bacteria on mum's skin and even on a baby's own skin as it discovers finger and toe sucking. Even as a baby breathes it takes in new bacteria. These bacteria quickly colonise the digestive tract and find a happy, warm and moist home in which to thrive and survive. Initially, within a few days, several types of bacteria will inhabit a baby's gut. Depending on the feeding method other bacteria will compete with these initial bacteria. This is healthy and necessary competition.

The gut flora of a formula fed baby is different from that of a breastfed baby. Breastfed babies tend to have a wider range of microbes in their gut than formula fed infants. We've known for some time that breastfeeding can provide many other health advantages for the baby but an understanding of the way in which breastfeeding may protect them by providing a more varied range of probiotics is fairly recent. An American study[11] revealed that breastfed babies are better able to absorb nutrients due to the boost in growth of gut flora. This is one possible explanation for some of the health benefits observed in breastfed babies.

TIME FROM BIRTH	BACTERIA	
1-2 DAYS	E.Coli, Enterobacteria, Enterococcus, Anerobes	
	Breast Fed	**Formula Fed**
1 WEEK	Lactobacilli and Bifidobacterium compete with initial bacteria to create balanced gut bacteria	Only Bifidobacterium start to compete. Lactobacilli are not present

Diet and gut bacteria

Changes to our diet can affect the type of gut bacteria we play host to. In one study[12] one particular species of gut bacteria called Akkermansia muciniphila, which lives in the mucus layer of the gut, was looked at in relation to dietary influences. It's a strain that's associated with being slimmer and better glucose tolerance in rodents. Except in this study the researchers wanted to see what happened in forty-nine overweight and obese adults when they followed a six-week calorie-restricted diet (between 1,500-1,800 calories per day) while increasing their fibre intake. The period of calorie restriction was followed by six weeks of eating normally.

The people who had more Akkermansia in their gut from the very start had better results after they completed the diet, compared to the people with less of the bacterium. Both groups of people lost the same amount of weight, but the group that had high levels of Akkermansia to begin with had a more marked reduction in visceral fat* than the others. This group also had a strong improvement in cholesterol, their ability to balance blood sugar levels, in waist to hip ratio and also a reduction in cardiovascular disease risk factors. Higher levels of Akkermansia, the findings suggest, seem to have favourable effects on multiple aspects of health.

*The type of fat that exists in the abdomen and surrounds the organs. Excessive deposits of visceral fat are associated with many serious health problems including cardiovascular disease, type 2 diabetes, and increased blood pressure.

Even people who had low levels of Akkermansia had significantly more after following the fibre-rich calorie-restricted diet than before. This means that increasing dietary fibre can have beneficial effects for everyone. Fibre is important to intestinal flora because gut microbes feed on it and produce short-chain fatty acids, which get absorbed into the bloodstream where they can regulate the immune system and reduce inflammation. The forms of fibre used in these experiments and the best forms of fibre for our overall health and wellbeing are those found in vegetables, nuts, seeds, whole grains and legumes.

When researchers replicate the typical Western diet* in mice, their gut microbes do something peculiar. They start eating away at the mucus lining of the intestine because this is a carbohydrate source, and for bacteria, the simplest form of energy. It is so far unclear whether the same thing happens in humans. However, if this is the case it could perhaps explain why bad diet, poor gut health and illness are often related.

In addition to the amount of Akkermansia we start with our ratios of firmicutes to bacteroidetes (the two main groups of bacteria found in humans and many other vertebrates) can also play a part in how our body responds to the foods we choose to eat and vice versa. Simply put, the foods we eat can change our ratios of bacteria. The reason these bacteria affect our weight is because they regulate how much fat we absorb. Imagine two identical twins eating exactly 2,000 calories, but they have different ratios of firmicutes to bacteroidetes. One will absorb more calories than the other and be more likely to gain weight on the exact same food, one 2008 study[13] suggested.

Multiple studies show that obese people have a higher concentration of firmicutes than bacteroidetes, whilst in lean people, the bacteroidetes predominate. A simple way to remember this is to think that fat and firmicutes both start with 'F', whilst beanpole and bacteroidetes begin with 'B'. However, studies have also shown that you can orchestrate a change in the ratio of microbiota you have through dietary intervention. Eating more polyphenols for example, a group of plant-based nutrients from brightly coloured fruit, vegetables, green tea and even coffee is linked to boosting the levels of bacteroidetes and supressing the growth of firmicutes.[14] A higher calorie diet seems to stimulate the growth of firmicutes. Whilst a high-fibre diet (from natural food sources including vegetables and other plant-based foods) can help reduce the number.

*A diet depleted of dietary fibre.

Sleeping patterns influence gut bacteria

Shift workers and frequent flyers are more likely to have a poorer balance of gut bacteria. Although this is a very recent area of study the findings are perhaps not surprising. Our gut bacteria operate according to a daily rhythm that we set by eating, sleeping and resting for consistent lengths of time. The body's microbiome adjusts to your own regular rhythm. However, the microbiota of those who work shifts or who travel to different time zones struggle to adjust and consequently, studies have shown an increase in an imbalance of gut bacteria that is linked to increased glucose intolerance and obesity[15].

In summary, the bacteria in our gut is influenced by many factors including our mother's diet, our birth method and how we are fed. It alters further over time, most likely due to dietary and environmental (including lifestyle) influences. It seems that many of these factors come together to increase or decrease the risk of developing obesity and ailments related to the immune system.[16]

Chapter 4

Meet Your Friends... an introduction to the good guys

There are lots of different types of bacteria calling your body home. It is worth investing some time in finding out a little more about these bacteria and how specific types may be able to improve specific areas of your health.

We often hear people refer to 'good' and 'bad' bacteria. Simplifying it this way we can say that the 'good' guys fall into four main categories:

1. Lactobacillus species	2. Bifidobacterium species	3. Saccharomyces species	4. Streptococcus species
L acidophilus	B bifidum	S boulardii	S thermophilus
L brevis	B infantis		S salivarius
L bulgaricus	B lactis		
L casei	B longum		
L reuteri	B breve		
L salivarius	B adolescentis		
L plantarum			
L fermentum			
L gasseri			
L johnsonii			
L lactis			
L paracasei			
L rhamnosus			

Each of the two main genera – lactobacillus and bifidobacterium - has multiple species such as lactis, brevis or breve. Their job description reads a little like this:

- Obtain the nutrients from the food eaten by your host to keep their body strong.
- Help the immune system in protecting your host against bacteria and viruses.

- Help the liver and kidneys to get rid of toxic substances.
- Keep the host's intestines healthy and strong and prevent inflammation in the gut as well as in other parts of the body.

There are several species receiving a lot of positive attention and research budgets right now in terms of disease prevention. They tend to have rather long and complicated names. However don't let this bamboozle you. These probiotic bacteria are so commonplace that many are simply floating in the air around you right now.

What's in a name?

Let's take an example of the probiotic **lactobacillus rhamnosus GG**. In order to work out what is being referred to let's break the name down into parts.

1. The first name is the **genus** (lactobacillus).
2. The second name designates the **species** within the genus (rhamnosus).
3. The third name or number that appears is the specific **strain** within the species (GG).

What makes things a little more confusing is when the names change. Lactobacillus GG (LGG) for example was initially classified as L. acidophilus strain GG, named after those that discovered it, Gorbach and Goldin. It was then named L.casei subspecies rhamnosum, or L. rhamnosum. More recently, scientists are arguing for it to be reclassified as a unique species, L. zeae. However, it is still commonly called Lactobacillus GG. These reclassifications and multiple names only cause problems when looking for research on specific strains and of course when trying to purchase them. If in doubt, then contact the manufacturer of the probiotic you are hoping to buy, to clarify.

Lactobacilli

These are the most widely researched probiotics and the name that most people who have ever purchased probiotic supplements will be familiar with. In fact, if you have a packet of probiotics in your house right now go and check the label. You'll notice that on the packet it will most likely refer to lactobacillus or perhaps this will have been abbreviated to L. Either way, this is the most common probiotic in both food and supplements. These bacteria are primarily found in the small intestine but are not limited to just this part of the body as you will also find them present in the upper respiratory tract, in the genital areas of both men and women and in the mucus membranes of the nose, mouth and throat. Large numbers of these bacteria are also found in the guts of pregnant women.

Lacobacillus bacteria produce lactic acid as their main product and also hydrogen peroxide (a natural antimicrobial which kills viruses, fungi and pathogenic bacteria.) They're tough fellows as they have to survive both stomach acid (the pH of which is as low as 1.5) and bile acid (the pH of which is as low as 2). They are naturally found in soil, vegetables, meat, milk and the human body. Many are in fermented foods such as yogurt, sauerkraut, traditionally pickled vegetables and kombucha. What I would advise is that rather than read this next section and think, 'ah that's the one probiotic strain for me,' keep an open mind. Not all research is carried out on individual strains and some strains are combined for both research purposes and useage, creating powerful combinations just as they exist in fermented foods as well as probiotic supplements. I would recommend these combinations as they have a significant amount of research to back their efficacy.

Studies have shown some benefits linked to lactobacillus and in terms of treating or preventing the following conditions:

Yeast infections, bacterial vaginosis (BV) and urinary tract infections (UTIs)

Candida albicans is a fungus. Whilst most people have some level of candida in their intestines, which usually co-exists peacefully with the other bacteria and yeasts that live there, some have a candida population that is out of control. When this is the case, it will establish fast growing colonies which will start to dominate the gut. When this happens a variety of symptoms including nausea, tiredness, sweet cravings, IBS, depression, allergies, palpitations, recurrent thrush and other fungal infections may occur. One particular probiotic supplement, L. paracasei, has been shown to reduce the rate of colonisation by candida albicans.[17] L. paracasei bacteria are typically found in dairy products such as live yogurt and kefir and they are also added to some infant formulas. You can also purchase L. paracasei supplements for therapeutic use. Other Lactobacillus strains have been shown to displace candida populations too. Lactobacillus strains are not alone when it comes to treating candida. They are often recommended in combination with other supplements to help restore optimal gut bacteria balance.

Certain Lactobacillus strains such as L. rhamnosus GR-1 and L. reuteri are shown to be the most effective in the prevention and treatment of recurrent urogenital infections, especially for recurrent bacterial vaginosis (BV). However, not all lactobacillus probiotics have shown such positive results. In fact, L. rhamnosus GG has not proved to be at all effective.

23

As to whether treatment with just probiotics would be superior to the antibiotic treatment, a 2013 study[18] from Bulgaria studied 381 women with bacterial vaginosis. The researchers split the patients into three groups. One group was given the probiotic treatment, the second group was given the antibiotic treatment and the third group was given a combination of both probiotics and antibiotics (the antibiotics were given first and followed by the probiotics). The researchers found there was a forty-three per cent success rate among the women who just took probiotics compared to a fifty-two per cent for those who had antibiotics. However, the best results were from the combined therapy, which had an eighty-seven per cent success rate. This of course means that the infection was knocked out by the antibiotics and then the gut microbes were restored by the probiotics. This is a powerful finding and it could inform the way in which doctors treat such infections and prevent them from reoccurring. Those suffering from B.V. would be wise not to take antibiotics alone if this is the treatment prescribed. Probiotics and antibiotics would be a preferred therapeutic treatment.

Irritable bowel syndrome (IBS)

In combination with several other specific species and strains of probiotics, certain lactobacillus species work to improve the symptoms of IBS. Improvements in aspects of IBS appear to be strain specific. In one study[19] pain associated with IBS reduced if the probiotic combinations contained B. breve, B. longum, or L. acidophilus species. In the same study, distention reduced if the probiotic combinations included B. breve and B.infantis as well as L.casei or L.plantarum, and flatulence lessened if the combination included B.breve, B.infantis, B.longum as well as L.casei, L.plantarum, L.acidophilus and L.bulgaricus, and Streptococcus salivarius ssp. thermophilus.

Further studies have revealed that the best probiotic for improving symptoms of IBS is L. plantarum. Results show that L. plantarum may decrease pain and flatulence in patients with IBS. The results of two studies[20, 21] suggest that supplementation in the short term with L.plantarum can have lasting effects.

One cause of IBS is lactose intolerance, a common digestive problem where the body is unable to digest lactose; a type of sugar mainly found in milk and dairy products. Various species of probiotics[22] have shown success in reducing the effects of lactose intolerance. There's also a well-known link between the bacteria found in yogurts and a reduction in the symptoms caused by the maldigestion of lactose.

Choosing the right supplement for symptoms of IBS can seem hard but trust good brands to get it right. The products that have the research to back their efficacy in treating the symptoms you suffer from most severely are worth paying for.

Improving skin health

Eczema is believed to be caused by a combination of genetic and environmental factors. Children are more likely to develop eczema if a parent has had it or another atopic disease*. If both parents have an atopic disease, the chances increase further. A very early study by probiotic research standards, from 2001, showed that children from families with a history of eczema found a benefit from probiotic supplementation. The researchers gave lactobacillus GG prenatally to mothers and postnatally for six months to their babies. The frequency of atopic eczema in the probiotic group was half that of the placebo group. This shows that the timely supplementation of lactobacillus GG in mothers and babies who have at least one first-degree relative (or partner) with atopic eczema, allergic rhinitis, or asthma could help reduce the risk of eczema developing. Both lactobacillus and bifidobacterium are both recommended for families at risk of atopic disease. Read on to find out how bifidobacterium bifidum has been shown to improve skin health too.

Rosacea is a skin condition characterised by redness and small, acne-like bumps on the face, and is often accompanied by red, watery eyes. Acne is a condition characterised by red bumps or pimples on the skin, especially the face. Antibiotics are often a treatment prescribed for both rosacea and acne. It is thought that the antibiotics may disrupt the normal microbial balance of the gut which is why probiotics may be able to undo some of the damage. Certainly studies seem to support this concept. In an Italian study[23], for example, half of the twenty adults with acne were administered an oral probiotic supplement in addition to their standard treatment. The other half of patients did not receive the probiotic supplement. The probiotic group experienced better clearing of symptoms. It's thought that the probiotics helped normalise skin expression which it is thought helped normalise skin expression of genes involved in the control of sugar. sugar. Probiotics are rarely thought of as a solution for rosacea and yet studies show they should be seriously considered. Whilst antibiotics are often prescribed to acne sufferers, alternative treatment and certainly the inclusion of gut balance restoring probiotics should also be considered.

Reducing cholesterol

Too much cholesterol in the blood can increase your risk of developing heart and circulatory diseases. Cholesterol is carried in the blood attached to proteins called lipoproteins. There are two main forms, LDL (low density lipoprotein) and HDL (high density lipoprotein). LDL cholesterol is often referred to as 'bad' cholesterol because too much is unhealthy. HDL is

*An atopic disease is a genetically inherited allergy like asthma, eczema or rhinitis

often referred to as 'good' cholesterol because it is protective. The probiotic L. Reuteri has been shown to reduce molecules known as cholesterol ester saturated fatty acids, which have been tied to dangerous plaque build-up in the arteries. In one particular study[24] people taking the probiotic L. Reuteri had total cholesterol reduced by 9.1 per cent and LDL cholesterol reduced by 11.6 per cent versus those on a placebo. HDL cholesterol and blood triglycerides, a dangerous form of fat in the blood, were unchanged. Other studies[25] have since been undertaken which only seem to substantiate L.Reuteri's role in reducing cholesterol.

The role of the probiotic L.Fermentum is also important[26]. This probiotic has been shown in multiple clinical studies to provide increased antioxidant activity and to improve the composition of the low-density lipid particles (LDL). One of the biggest concerns with high cholesterol is atherosclerosis (an artery that gets blocked by fatty substances called plaques) L. Reuteri and L. Fermentum both seem to provide beneficial effects for those at risk of both high cholesterol and atherosclerosis. Probiotic supplementation should support dietary intervention in the treatment of cholesterol and the prevention of atherosclerosis.

Reducing inflammation

Gut-associated inflammation has been linked to insulin-resistance, some forms of cancer and mental health issues. The role of probiotics in the treatment of inflammation is to outcompete the bacteria causing the inflammation. The probiotic L. Brevis has been shown to help in the treatment of periodontitis which is a form of inflammation.[28] It's a disease that causes loosening of the teeth in the gums. This is an important finding as more people suffer from inflammation related illnesses than ever before. Inflammatory markers are tested using a simple blood test which is available from your doctor. Raised levels of inflammatory markers can be caused by infections, autoimmune conditions, and certain cancers. This is an early area of study for many researchers but the impact of inflammation on health is not in any doubt. Therefore the role of probiotics in reducing inflammation needs also to be considered. This could be approached through specific supplementation treatment plans and/or through the inclusion of fermented (probiotic) foods in the regular diet of those suffering from inflammation.

Preventing MRSA

With the rise in antibiotic resistant strains of certain pathogenic bacteria the worldwide medical community might well look to probiotics to prevent infection. One such resistant, pathogenic bacterium is methicillin-resistant S. aureus, otherwise known as MRSA. Research has shown that L. paracasei could act as a potential barrier to prevent S. aureus- associated illness[29]. This probiotic strain produced a bacteriocin like substance (a substance produced by bacteria to stop the growth of similar or closely related bacterial strains) active against the staphylococcal strains. This is not the only probiotic to show positive outcomes in the prevention of MRSA. Probiotics must be considered for use in hospitals and other clinical settings.

Suppressing Helicobactor pylori

Helicobacter pylori are one of the most common bacteria in the stomach. We are not born with these bacteria but we pick them up from our environment as children. Many people have no symptoms associated with H.Pylori infection. However, the spiral shape of the bacteria and the way in which they move allows them to penetrate the stomach's protective mucus lining, weakening it and making the stomach more vulnerable to gastric acids. In those people who are more susceptible to the effects of H.Pylori the bacteria can stimulate the production of excess stomach acid, which can lead to gastritis (inflammation of the stomach). In fact, the majority of ulcers in the stomach and all ulcers in the small intestine can be attributed to H.Pylori. Infection with the bacteria is also associated with a very slight increase in the risk of stomach cancer too. Although intriguingly, it seems that simply having H.Pylori present may offer protective benefits against other cancers and also childhood asthma. The probiotic L. Gasseri has been shown to be effective in multiple studies in both supressing H.Pylori and reducing symptoms or, in combination with antibiotic therapy, of eradicating it[30]. Medical professionals provide a fairly standard drug focused solution to H.Pylori infections currently. The evidence suggests that probiotics should also be considered as part of the treatment of this health condition.

Addressing diabetes

Studies show differences in the composition of the gut microbiota between children with type 1 diabetes and those without. Children with diabetes are found to have greatly decreased numbers of the 'good' bacteria lactobacillus, bifidobacterium and Prevotella. This is significant because scientists also found that a higher number of bifidobacterium and lactobacillus co-exists with better blood sugar control[31].

Another group scientists studied thirty-three infants from Finland who were all genetically predisposed to Type 1 Diabetes. They found that four of the infants had twenty-five per cent less variation of bacteria in their guts compared to other children. These four were also found to have more of specific bacteria associated with inflammation. Type 1 diabetes is an autoimmune condition in which bacteria causes the immune system to mistakenly attack and destroy beta cells in the pancreas that help balance glucose levels. The lack of gut bacteria and associated inflammatory bacteria could help explain why this autoimmune response takes place[32].

This health condition might not have an obvious relationship with gut health and yet we are now finding out that the two are intrinsically linked. The question is if a lack of 'good' bacteria is part of the problem then can probiotics be part of the solution. Put simply, can probiotics improve sensitivity to insulin? The answer appears to be yes. The exact mechanism seems to be related to probiotics getting gut cells to behave more like the pancreatic cells of healthy people which help to regulate blood sugar levels.

The possible effect of probiotics on type 2 diabetic patients is different. Probiotics have anti-inflammatory properties and the insulin resistance in type 2 diabetes is associated with chronic inflammation. So the anti-inflammatory actions of probiotics increase sensitivity to insulin, which is turn helps to manage glucose (sugar) levels in the body. One probiotic that may have a treatment role in the management of this disease is L. johnsonii. One 2006 study[33] found that the oral administration of L. johnsonii reduced both glucose and glucagon (which is released in response to low blood glucose therefore playing the opposite role to insulin) levels in diabetic rats which had been subject to an injection into the brain of glucose.

In another study, L. Rhamnosus improved a number of markers including blood sugar balance, triglycerides, cholesterol, and oxidative stress in rats with diabetes[34]. The results of the studies are promising. With time and greater testing on humans with type 2 diabetes we should know if probiotics are a viable, additional treatment option.

Preventing Illness

Not only do probiotics have a role to play in treating illness when it occurs but lactobacillus in particular may also help to prevent health problems. One such illness is salmonellosis which is an infection caused by the bacteria salmonella. The bacteria can be picked up from food or water that has become contaminated. Symptoms include fever, headache, diarrhoea and vomiting. In several studies, the probiotic L.salivarius has been shown to reduce the incidence of salmonella both in chickens[35] which of course will then enter the food chain to be consumed by humans, but also in horses[36] which suffer from the effects of salmonella too and this probiotic has been shown to help reduce the incidence of gastrointestinal problems. Let us not forget that the lower part of our gut is rather like that of a horse. These two studies provide clues as to how this probiotic strain could be used to reduce the incidence of gastrointestinal problems in humans as a result of food poisoning in the first place.

Probiotics have also proved to be effective in the prevention of antibiotic associated diarrhoea and Clostridium difficile associated diarrhoea among adults in hospital. This conclusion was drawn from a meta-analysis of eight studies including 1,246 participants, on the effect of probiotics on either antibiotic-associated diarrhoea or C. Difficile[37]. Both MRSA and C. Difficile are such a prevalent threat to hospital patients. Results of research on probiotics suggest that both could be prevented or reduced by probiotic intervention.

Lactobacillus bacteria have also been shown to ward off various pathogens. A 2017 study[38] showed how effective L. reuteri strains are in this capacity. It appears that lactobacillus bacteria not only help to prevent or address specific health issues, by protecting the body from pathogens, they have a leading role in disease prevention.

Bifidobacteria

These bacteria are most commonly found in the mouth, the GI tract, the large intestine, and in the vagina. Just as the lactobacillus is abbreviated to L., bifidobacteria is abbreviated to B. Also just like lactobacillus, their function varies from species to species. However, there are about seven times as many bifidobacterium as lactobacilli in the gut of a healthy adult. Although they are less well researched than lactobacillus, the research that has been carried out so far is exciting in terms of how relevant to prevention or reduction of disease the use of these probiotics may become. Here's what bifidobacterium are capable of, either as an individual species or in combination with other probiotics and prebiotics.

Reducing allergic (including histamine) reactions -

Bifidobacterium bifidum has been found to increase antibodies IgG, IgM and IgA and discourage the production of histamine in food allergy[39]. A study[40] combining multiple bifidobacterium and lactobacillus strains found that treatment with this mixture could decrease anaphylaxis scores. Allergic individuals taking this probiotic had decreased levels of histamine in their stools, when compared to those who had not taken the mix. This was associated with a reduction in tissue levels of inflammatory cytokines* and an increase in the tissue levels of regulatory cytokines. These studies show promise in the administration of probiotics to humans with food allergies.

Other research looks at the use of probiotics as a delivery mechanism for genetically modified versions of the allergic foods to particular areas within the gastrointestinal tract. The idea behind this is that when those with food

---

*Cytokines are cell signalling molecules that aid cell to cell communication in immune responses and stimulate the movement of cells towards sites of inflammation, infection and trauma.

allergies are exposed to the unmodified versions of the food, they do not react. With so many people, in particular children, suffering with life-threatening food allergy, this is a promising area of research indeed. In fact, several studies have explored this way of using probiotics with positive results.[41, 42]

Addressing skin health

The link between skin health and gut health is being understood more and more. One of the most common findings is that bifidobacterium bifidum helps to reduce inflammation and irritation in patients with eczema[43]. Also bifidobacterium strains in combination with lactobacillus strains have been proven successful in reducing eczema symptoms.

Bifidobacterium infantis is typically found in the digestive system of babies and rarely in adults. Its role includes breaking down human milk for digestion and boosting the immune system. In this capacity, bifidobacterium infantis has been linked to reducing the inflammatory processes in another skin condition called psoriasis, an autoimmune condition where skin cells reproduce too quickly, resulting in a build-up of skin cells[44]. Choosing a multi-strain probiotic containing at least Lactobacillus GG and Bifidobacterium Bifidum is advised for mothers and babies at risk from atopic diseases.

Improving coeliac symptoms

Coeliac disease mostly affects the small intestine. It is caused by a reaction of the gut to gluten, a protein contained within grains such as wheat, barley and rye. Studies have shown that people with coeliac disease have different microbes living in their intestines compared to people without the condition. A 2008 study[45] published in BMC Microbiology found reduced numbers of total bifidobacterium microbes in children with coeliac disease. The same study found higher levels of helpful bifidobacterium microbes in the children's intestines after they had begun a gluten free diet, suggesting that their microbiome may have begun to recover. However, the coeliac children still had lower levels than normal of the helpful microbes, even when on the diet. The results suggest that total and specific bifidobacterium species could be possible protective factors for coeliac disease. Therefore, the administration of specific probiotics to increase their levels could be a suitable additional therapeutic strategy for this condition.

One specific probiotic showing hope in this area is B. lactis bacteria which has been shown to counteract the harmful effects of gluten [46]. The way in which this appears to work can be explained by first understanding the effect of the gluten protein on intestinal cells. In those with coeliac disease, gluten activates an immune response among the intestinal cells which results in the secretion of a protein called zonulin. This stimulates an increase in the spaces in the tight junctions between the intestinal cells, creating leaky gut syndrome. This opening between intestinal cells is accompanied by an even greater inflammatory response as the immune system responds to larger proteins having contact with the bloodstream. There is now evidence of intestinal probiotics inhibiting this process by breaking down gluten through enzyme activity. The enzyme involved is called 'protease'.

Evidence points towards a positive outcome for coeliac sufferers from using probiotics to reduce the severity of their symptoms.

Beyond lactobacillus and bifidobacterium

Positive health benefits are not only associated with lactobacillus and bifidobacterium but also other beneficial microbes such as yeasts and in other bacterium too such as Streptococcus Thermophilus.

Sacchromyces boulardii (pronounced Sack-row-my-sees bu-lar-dee)

S. Bouladrii is a microorganism which differs greatly from the well-known probiotic species such as acidophilus. Saccharomyces boulardii is actually natural yeast. It was discovered by a Frenchman called Henri Boulard who patented it as an anti-diarrhoea drug - S. boulardii (as it can also be written). It provides benefits for the gastrointestinal tract in a variety of ways. It makes bacterial toxins inactive, stops toxins from sticking the gastrointestinal tract and reduces inflammation caused by toxins. S. boulardii stimulates our immune defences and the enzymes that improve digestion and absorption rates. It produces acids that combat potentially harmful microorganisms, assists in mineral absorption and nourishes the colon. It has been tested and verified by scientists as an anti-microbial that can benefit humans suffering from C. difficile, E. coli and candida overgrowth. This microorganism is understood to be a transient. That means that it passes through the system without binding to the gut wall lining. S. boulardii provides a useful reminder that not all yeast is bad, far from it. This particular yeast is good for people with suffering from diarrhoea or gastroenteritis.

Streptococcus thermophilus

The probiotic Streptococcus thermophilus is a starter culture in the manufacturing process of yogurt, mozzarella cheese and other fermented dairy products. One of the principal therapeutic uses for S. thermophilus is for the relief of the abdominal cramps, diarrhoea, nausea and other gastrointestinal symptoms associated with lactose intolerance.

Streptococcus salivarius

Given that one of the causes of halitosis (the medical term for bad breath) is an imbalance of gut bacteria it makes sense that the use of a probiotic may improve symptoms. The probiotic Streptococcus salivarius has been shown to do just this[49]. The mechanism by which the bacteria works is by reducing the presence of the halitosis causing bacteria, by crowding them out of the gut.

What you can take from all of these examples is an overwhelming message that probiotics can be a very useful part of an overall strategy to prevent ill health and promote wellbeing as well as specifically addressing some health problems. As suggested earlier, you should be wary of assuming the 'pill for an ill' mentality and assuming that one strain of probiotic is suitable for your specific health problem. Rather, probiotics should be used as part of an overall strategy and should be taken in combination, not only with other probiotics but also with other therapies and lifestyle changes.

Chapter 5

Which Gut Type Are You?

In much the same way as scientists mapped the human genome, so they are now trying to map the human microbiome. They have discovered that we are made up of more than ten thousand microbial species and that the microbiome consists of 8 million protein coding genes which you'd think would make for a lot of possible permutations when it comes to gut types. Yet a new area of our understanding of the gut and the microbiome is based on the possibility that we may all fall into groups or 'gut types', also known as enterotypes. In 2011, scientists came up with a hypothesis that we humans could be categorised into one of three types, according to our gut microbiomes[50]. These gut types are based on there being a predominant bacteria present in each. Each enterotype does things slightly differently.

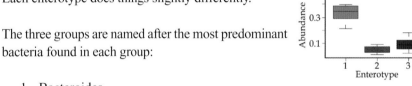

The three groups are named after the most predominant bacteria found in each group:

1. Bacteroides
2. Prevotella
3. Ruminococcus

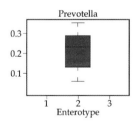

Scientists do not yet have a conclusive explanation for why these three groups of gut microbiota exist. In fact, some camps even refute their existence. However, one possibility is that the guts of babies are randomly colonised by different pioneering species of microbes. The microbes alter the gut so that only certain species can follow them; so the initial bacteria set up the host and then dictate which other bacteria are attracted to colonise. Knowing and understanding the differences between the three types could be very helpful in terms of identifying the best course of preventative medicine or lifestyle changes for particular individuals.

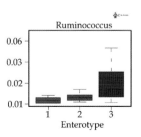

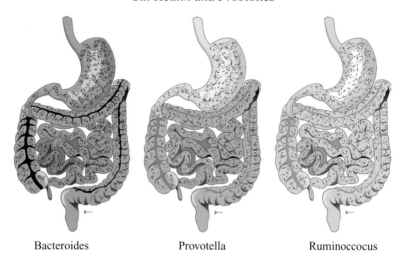

| Bacteroides | Provotella | Ruminoccocus |

Relationship to BMI

The body mass index (BMI) is a measure that uses your height and weight to work out if you have a healthy body mass. Investigations into these three gut types show that there is a correlation between body mass index (BMI) and the strains of bacteria in each enterotype. The more efficiently the bacteria can take out the calories (energy) from the food consumed, the greater the chance that the person has a higher BMI and therefore the greater the chance they may struggle with their weight. Ruminococcus, for example, is commonly associated with weight gain because it helps cells to absorb sugar. Those whose predominant bacteria are bacteroides tend to be leaner. The identification of gut type could be used in the future as a predictor of obesity. With this knowledge interventions could be made to limit the chances of people becoming obese.

Differences in vitamin production

Gut microbes help food to be digested and to extract vitamins using enzymes our own cells cannot make. The research so far has found that each of the three identified enterotypes makes a unique balance of these enzymes. Bacteroides produce more enzymes for making vitamins C, B2, B5 and vitamin B7 (also known as biotin), for example, and Prevotella make more enzymes for vitamin B1 (thiamine) and vitamin B9 (folic acid). This knowledge of an individual's gut type could inform nutrient supplementation programmes.

Dietary influence on the three groups

Whilst the Bacteroides enterotype is more associated with urban dwellers, the Prevotella enterotype is associated with people who live in more rural areas[51]. In studies of these three enterotypes, it was found that people who ate predominantly meat and saturated fats had more Bacteroides than those who ate a fibre-rich and plant-based diet who had higher levels of Provotella, perhaps reflecting the predominant foodstuffs available in each environment. However, Ruminococcus was the most predominant and there was a definite link between this group and the ample consumption of alcohol and polyunsaturated fats.

Differences between the three groups

Multiple studies show that being from a particular enterotype may have benefits in terms of health markers. For example, those from the Prevotella group tend to have lower LDL cholesterol levels [52] and this enterotype provides immunity to diarrhoea, actively helping children in poorer African communities[53]. Yet, studies also show that people in the Prevotella group with rheumatoid arthritis have worse symptoms, than those with other enterotypes[54].

Why is this useful research?

Knowing which enterotype a person is could have real implications for personalised medicine, in which treatments can be tailored to an individual's needs. We already know, for example, that gut bacteria help in metabolising drugs and change the absorption behaviour of human cells. It's likely that the three enterotypes do this in different ways, so optimal dosage of medicine (and balance of food) might be different for each one. At present, the type of medication given and the dosage administered is not based on a person's gut type. It is most likely to be focused on the particular ailment and the patient's body mass. Knowing a person's entertotype may lead to more bespoke medication and supplementation plans and reduction in the prescription of unnecessary medication.

Is it possible to change your gut type?

Many studies have shown dramatic shifts in microbiome diversity after very short periods of dietary change. Dietary intervention such as increasing the amounts of fibre in the diet, reducing reliance on overly processed foods and decreasing sugars combined with an increased consumption of probiotic foods or supplements have been shown to dramatically improve gut bacteria status and prevalence amongst subjects in multiple studies. One such study in 2014[55] concluded that 'dietary habits may be the most important contributing factor to changes in enterotype status'. The speed at which microbiota could be changed by dietary intervention suggest this is a very useful strategy for improving overall health and health markers.

In summary, the existence of enterotypes is an exciting finding but certainly one that requires more definition. Further research and a deeper understanding of these groups could prove to be really useful in terms of prescriptions, supplementation plans and recommendations for longer term dietary changes.

Chapter 6

When a Good Neighbourhood Turns Bad!

The term 'dysbiosis' was first used by Dr Eli Metchnikoff in the early 1920s. It is derived from two words, 'symbiosis' meaning living together in harmony, and 'dis' which means not. Metchnikoff used this word to describe a microbial imbalance within the intestines. Today we comprehend just how powerful an understanding of dysbiosis may be in the treatment of disease. It took some time for the medical profession to make a connection between microbial imbalance and disease. Once the connection was made, however, scientists discovered links between poor gut health and numerous diseases, many not actually associated with the intestines. The consistent factor linking poor health and dysbiosis seems to be inflammation and this provides many clues as to how addressing dysbiosis may also address health problems.

Once dysbiosis is established, harmful intestinal flora start to act on the gut. Dysbiosis may be caused by, but is certainly characterised by putrefaction, fermentation, nutrient deficiency and sensitivity to allergens. The number of inflammatory diseases within the bowel or involving the skin and connective tissue that have been reported in association with dysbiosis is growing as our understanding of the importance of this imbalance grows.

Although the health of the gut is in part already predetermined by your mother's diet, the way you entered the world and were fed in your earliest days, it is thought that people do actually play a part in creating their own state of dysbiosis. It is evident that dietary and lifestyle choices play a huge role in the potential for dysbiosis to develop. Stress, medication, diet and the living environment all have their part to play but is there perhaps another explanation?

'...death sits in the bowels...' Hippocrates 400 B.C.

Your body attacks healthy gut flora

Autoimmune diseases such as rheumatoid arthritis, lupus, MS, coeliac disease and ankylosing spondylitis have already been linked to dysbiosis. In determining

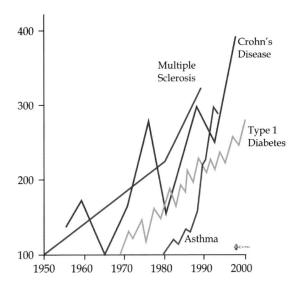

Incidence of autoimmune disorders from 1950 to 2000.

the cause of dysbiosis there is quite a lot of evidence to suggest that the body attacks its own healthy gut flora. In the last forty years, there has been a realisation that exaggerated immune responses to normal gut bacteria are possible causes of inflammatory bowel diseases such as Crohn's disease and ulcerative colitis[56]. In cases such as these the obvious question is what leads the body to launch an autoimmune reaction in the first place? Recent insight in to this has been offered by a 2017 study[57] which suggests a case of misidentification on the part of the immune system of dysbiotic individuals. The healthy human gut contains bacteria that can secrete a substance that helps to create barriers and stable structures; this is a helpful and healthy product of symbiotic bacteria. However, if this substance is secreted by bacteria in a dysbiotic gut this can cause the body to confuse its own gut cells for these dysbiotic cells and attack them. This appears to happen through some form of molecular mimicry. However, it is unclear whether the autoimmune response triggers the dysbiosis or the dysbiosis triggers the autoimmune disease. Certainly, what is clear is that the number of people with autoimmune diseases has increased dramatically in the past sixty years. What's more is that autoimmunity does seem to be a Western problem. That alone should make us curious as to the cause.

Low stomach acid and dysbiosis

The stomach is lined with cells that are proton pumps - that is to say they pump hydrogen ions from the bloodstream into the stomach. Stomach acid is simply concentrated hydrogen ions. There is a natural tendency for these hydrogen ions to diffuse back to where they came from but this is prevented by very tight junctions between stomach wall cells. However, if the gut becomes inflamed for whatever reason, leaky gut can develop and hydrogen ions leak back out. Low stomach acid can manifest itself as a multitude of digestive issues including wind, gas, bloating as foods become fermented and not digested and the poor absorption of nutrients (an acidic environment is required for effective absorption). Low stomach acid is not only a natural outcome it can be precipitated by use of particular medications. Antacids are an obvious culprit for reducing stomach acid for example but stress, age, a diet high in refined carbohydrates, a diet low in protein, hormone changes and certain surgeries are also to blame.

While a common cause of dysbiosis is low stomach acid levels, it is also a common symptom. This can lead to bacterial overgrowth in the gut as the PH of the gut becomes more alkaline, creating a very different environment for bacteria to live in. This allows pathogenic (disease causing) bacteria to flourish whilst those good bacteria that are part of the immune defence are unable to do their job properly.

Stress and dysbiosis

Chronic (long-term) stress elevates 'stress' hormones which also wreak havoc on your immunity, making you more susceptible to an imbalance of gut bacteria. Research has found that exposure to stress leads to an overgrowth of certain types of bacteria while simultaneously reducing the range of microbes in the large intestine[58]. One study found a reduction in the levels of lactobacillus and an increase in circulating kynurenine levels (higher levels have been linked to depression) as the most prominent changes when under stress. Restoring intestinal lactobacillus levels improves mood. The lactobacillus plays a role in keeping kynurenine levels in check. If lactobacillus is too low then levels of kynurenine are allowed to rise and that means a greater probability of depression.

We know that psychological stress can have an effect on gastrointestinal and digestive secretions by lowering the amounts produced for digestion purposes, changing the way food is passed through the digestive system, slowing the process down and allowing putrefaction and fermentation to take place. Furthermore, stress causes a reduction in the substances that stop pathogens from sticking to the gut lining. It has been proven that under stressful conditions we produce less secretory IgA, which is part of our immune defence against pathogens looking to colonise our gut. Secretory IgA plays a vital role in both protecting the gastrointestinal tract from the colonisation of bad bacteria but also in reducing the levels too.

'...bad digestion is the root of all evil....' Hippocrates 400 B.C.

Medication and dysbiosis

The use of antibiotics, birth control, painkillers and steroids can make people particularly susceptible to dysbiosis. They cause damage to the intestinal lining, which in turn causes more inflammation, irritation and pain. The result is that we take more pain medication which causes further damage.

One of the more common medications for pain relief is a combination of cortisone and prednisone. These corticosteroids, as they are known, have a very powerful anti-inflammatory effect on the body. As a result, they tend to be used long-term by people with chronic illness. However, there is a downside. The long-term use of corticosteroids depresses the intestinal immune system, which means it is unable to fight back when pathogens enter the body. They're also not advised for people suffering from fungal infections as they provide fuel allowing fungi to thrive.

Many people also rely on non-steroidal anti-inflammatory drugs (NSAIDs such as Ibuprofen) for pain relief. These drugs inhibit the growth of healthy bacteria in the gut. Research shows that chronic exposure to NSAIDs produces a state of leaky gut, associated with inflammation, which seems to be both prevented and reversed by the administration of the antibiotic, metronidazole[59]. This course of treatment provides big clues as to the importance of bacterial toxins in maintaining this vicious cycle. It makes one wonder if probiotic treatment would not be a more suitable partner to NSAIDs to prevent intestinal permeability associated with the use of these painkillers.

The most common prescription medicine causing dysbiosis is antibiotics, possibly explaining why dysbiosis is such a Western problem. Viral illnesses are commonly treated with antibiotics, and while this may be effective in dealing with an acute bacterial infection, these so-called wide spectrum antibiotics kill off a large range of bacteria, including the normal healthy bugs in the gut. This is why abnormal bowel action, particularly diarrhoea, commonly follows a course of antibiotics. Ironically, the overuse of antibiotics increases the need for future antibiotics, as the dysbiosis induced by them suppresses the immune system and allows for further bacterial infection.

Hormones in the form of hormone elevating drugs, including birth control, menopause treatments and steroid hormones, can all spark an imbalance of gut flora. In turn, this can lead to invasion by pathogenic bacteria or an overgrowth of fungus or yeast. Many people who are prescribed hormone medication such as the contraceptive pill will notice symptoms associated with bacterial or yeast overgrowth such as Candida albicans start to emerge after a period on the medication.

Environment and dysbiosis

Living in a damp, foggy climate, the presence of mould or fungus in the home, and exposure to toxic chemicals and metals can increase susceptibility to dysbiosis. Travelling abroad where exposure to contaminated water and food is more likely has been linked to an increase likelihood of dysbiosis. Recent research[60] has highlighted the possible link between dysbiosis and Parkinson's disease. It seems that people exposed to high levels of pesticides and who drink from wells are more likely to suffer from Parkinson's. This suggests there could be a link between chemical exposure of Parkinson's sufferers and a change to their gut microbiota. Furthermore, the overuse of pesticides, the overuse of antibiotics in farming and the consequent run-off into the waterways that feed into human water supplies are all thought to be contributing to greater dysbiosis rates in humans.

Eating habits and dysbiosis

In spite of the way we are nurtured in our mother's wombs, and in spite of the way we enter the world there are still some elements of our own choices in life that determine the overall health of our microbiome. Not least is what we choose to eat. For example, a diet very low in soluble fibre may create deficiency of normal gut bacteria, including bifidobacteria, lactobacillus and E. Coli. These bacteria are often found to be low in stool tests on patients with irritable bowel syndrome and food intolerances. Diets high in processed food, in particular processed forms of protein and food additives, have been shown to contribute greatly to the production of potentially toxic products through gut fermentation. Let's take a look at a typical day's food intake to try to understand where we may be going wrong in the Western world.

TYPICAL DAY'S FOOD INTAKE:	
Breakfast	'Skinny' latte, cinnamon raisin bagel
Lunch	Filled baguette – chicken & salad 0% fat strawberry yogurt Diet cola
Mid-Afternoon Snack	Chocolate rice cakes and tea
Evening Meal	Pasta with oven roasted vegetables and goat's cheese, large glass of wine

Although typical of the modern Western diet, this kind of intake actually reflects the food decisions of people who believe they are making better, healthier choices. Yet, these are not optimal choices for a healthier biome. Let's understand why:

1. Mostly food choices are based on a general belief that low fat is better for our health as well as our long term wellbeing. In actual fact, once you take the fat out of a food that naturally contains fat, the sugar level often increases in order to make the food palatable. For example, a plain, fat free yogurt free natural yogurt contains approximately 7.5g of sugar per 100g of product. While a plain Greek yogurt yogurt contains about 5g of

sugar per 100g. So in pursuit of low fat we could end up consuming more sugars. Added to this, some fats can actually boost gut bacteria diversity and reduce inflammation. These are the omega 3 fats found in wild oily fish, seeds and their oils and certain nuts. The majority of people in the western world eat too few omega 3 foods.

2. Whilst many people choose to eat lower calorie foods, a lack of nutrient-dense foods can reduce the diversity of the gut microbiome which we will discover can be linked to poor health and even weight gain. That's not to say that the two things are mutually exclusive but by focussing mostly on calorie consumption people often eat processed foods with a nutrition label rather than nutrient-dense foods without a nutrition label so they can control their calorie consumption.

3. The modern Western diet contains a lot of wheat. If every meal is based on a carbohydrate choice of wheat there's a great deal of monotony and therefore a lack of nutrient diversity. This lack of diversity can be mirrored in a lack of diverse gut bacteria too. Furthermore, a lot of wheat is sprayed with the herbicide glyphosate which works by disrupting a pathway specific to gut bacteria. Until recently, it was thought that no harm to humans could be caused by glyphosate. Now that we understand that the same pathway that is disrupted in plants may also be disrupted in human gut bacteria too, we understand how modern wheat may be causing some people to have gut problems.

4. Although there are some vegetables in this set of meal choices this certainly wouldn't make up 5-a-day portions and now the latest research suggests we should be aiming for at least 7-a-day. This is just a dream for many eating a standard Western diet. Yet an abundance of vegetables means more vegetable fibres. Vegetable fibres are the very substance that feeds the good bacteria in the large intestine.

5. Diet cola is sweetened with artificial sweeteners. These have been shown to alter gut bacteria. A team of Israeli scientists concluded from research that ingesting artificial sweeteners might lead to obesity and conditions like diabetes[61]. This study was not the first to note this link, but it was the first to find evidence of a plausible cause. It seems that the sweeteners appear to change the population of intestinal bacteria that are in turn responsible for aiding the process of metabolism (the conversion of food to energy or to stored energy).

Our modern diet is far higher in sugar than our bodies are designed to handle. What we have learnt from many years of study is that bacteria thrive on sugar. It is a simple form of fuel, easily converted into energy and used for their survival. If our digestive system is working as it was intended then most of the sugar consumed in the form of food and drink would have been absorbed by the time it reaches the colon. However it seems that the majority of us do not have a perfectly functioning digestive system.

In summary, although we are born into this world with a range of gut bacteria which is determined by our mother's microbiome, the way we arrived in the world (birthing method) and the way in which we were fed in those early days, the decisions we make for ourselves, even as we become adults, can have a huge influence on the microbiome and the balance or imbalance of bacteria to be found there. From the environment we live in, to the chemicals we are exposed to, the medication we take and the food we eat, all these factors play a part in the level of dysbiosis we have in our gastrointestinal tract.

Chapter 7

Dysbiosis and Disease

Dysbiosis weakens our ability to protect ourselves from disease. There is growing evidence that dysbiosis of the gut is associated with the occurrence of both intestinal and extraintestinal disorders. Intestinal disorders include inflammatory bowel disease such as Crohn's disease and ulcerative colitis, irritable bowel syndrome (IBS), and coeliac disease, while extraintestinal disorders include allergies, asthma, metabolic syndrome (pre-diabetes), cardiovascular disease, obesity as well as mental health issues.

It is acknowledged that the presence of abnormal bacteria in the gastrointestinal tract can result in:

- Deactivation of digestive enzymes that can lead to poor digestion and absorption - and ultimately malnutrition
- Reduced absorption of vitamin B12 and certain amino acids [62]
- Disruption of the intestinal lining that can cause leaky gut syndrome[63]
- Development of yeast/fungi overgrowth, parasite infection or allow pathogenic bacteria to thrive
- Development of irritable bowel syndrome and inflammatory bowel disease

Let's take a look at some of the evidence of dysbiosis being related to specific diseases.

Disease	Evidence of dysbiosis
Atopic Eczema	According to a recent study, in the majority of cases, atopic eczema sufferers had evidence of small bowel dysbiosis and malabsorption[64].
Irritable Bowel Syndrome (IBS)	Stool testing revealed that patients suffering from irritable bowel syndrome have abnormal gut bacteria[65].

Disease	Evidence of dysbiosis
Inflammatory Bowel Disease (IBD)	People with Crohn's disease and ulcerative colitis tend have less 'good' bacteria in their gut and less diversity. Specifically, they have lower levels of Firmicutes and an increase in Bacteroidetes and also potentially pathogenic bacteria such as Enterobacteriaceae[66]. Bacterial overgrowth of the jejunum has been found in 30% of patients hospitalised for Crohn's disease, in which it contributes to diarrhoea and malabsorption[67]. Increased prevalence of leaky gut syndrome in patients with active Crohn's disease and in healthy first degree relatives suggests the existence of a pre-existing gut health issue that results in an exaggerated immune response [68].
Arthritis and Ankylosing Spondylitis	Intestinal infections Yersinia and Salmonella have been linked to reactive arthritis[69], while patients with ankylosing spondylitis have been found to have higher levels of Klebsiella pneumoniae in their stools and higher levels of anti-Klebsiella IgA in their blood. [70]

As a result of dysbiosis, various pathogens are allowed to thrive in our intestinal tracts. They range from parasites to viruses and fungi to bacteria. While some of these 'visitors' are already welcome in our gastrointestinal tract in smaller numbers, the presence of dysbiosis gives them an opportunity to replicate and to multiply to levels that cause ill health. Other visitors are then opportunistic and enter the gastrointestinal tract while the host is in a weakened immune state. The unwanted visitors include:

Small Bacteria Intestinal Overgrowth (SIBO)

Bacteria exist throughout the digestive tract. However the levels of bacteria in the small intestine are normally relatively low. An overgrowth of bacteria in the small intestine may be the result of slower movement of food through the digestive system which could result from a variety of preceding conditions.

Reasons for SIBO
Low thyroid function
Coeliac disease
Stress
Medication, including immunosuppressant's and proton pump inhibitors
Diabetes
Age

Symptoms of SIBO
Gas and Flatulence
Bloating
Malabsorption of nutrients
Rosacea
Fibromyalgia
IBS

Parasites

Of all of the potential growths in our guts, the one that people are most disgusted by is parasites. By definition, a parasite is a living organism that survives within a host but at the expense of that host. In the case of the human gut, a parasite can cause a variety of symptoms as your immune system reacts to an unwanted invader. Parasites known to infect the human gut include worms and single-celled organisms. It's a lot easier than people think to pick up parasites too.

Sources of parasite infection:
1) Water/food contamination
2) Overseas travel
3) Sexual partners
4) Pets

Your doctor may not realise you have a parasite, even if you have various different health issues. Here are some of the most common symptoms of a parasite infection:

Symptoms of parasite infection:
1) Abdominal pain, nausea/vomiting, constipation/diarrhea
2) Joint and muscle aches
3) Skin rashes, eczema
4) Chronic pain
5) Fatigue
6) Itching
7) Unexplained fever
8) Unexplained weight loss

Fungi

Although many yeasts and fungi exist within our natural gut environment, problems arise when they overgrow and cause symptoms. This can happen when immune defences are lowered as a result of diet, stress or medication, often in combination with a toxin overload.

Sources of fungal infection:
1) Antibiotics
2) Steroid use (Prednisone, etc.), including steroid inhalers
3) Birth control pills and hormone replacement therapy may contribute to the problem, but may not be enough to cause the problem on their own. This is less common with bioidentical hormones as it is with synthetic hormones.
4) Mould exposure (via inhalation or skin contact) through workplace, home, etc.
5) Hot, humid environments (contribute to mould formation/exposure)
6) Sexual partner (exchange of saliva can be enough to spread infection in susceptible individuals)

Symptoms of fungal infection:
1) Fatigue
2) Brain fog
3) Abdominal symptoms, such as nausea, vomiting, constipation, diarrhoea, bloating and flatulence
4) GERD (reflux)
5) Depression, mood swings, and other psychiatric conditions
6) Migraines and headaches
7) Skin rashes, eczema, psoriasis
8) Asthma, respiratory problems
9) Yeast infection of skin, mouth and vagina
10) Chemical sensitivities

Viruses

When we think of viruses, most of us think of colds and respiratory infections. However, there are many different types of viruses that can cause a wide range of symptoms, some of them deadly. Viruses are transmitted via the nose, mouth or breaks in the skin. Although viruses are smaller than bacteria their power lies in their ability to replicate rapidly once in the body. They do this through a process called the 'lytic cycle'. This is where the virus reproduces itself using

Replica cycle of a virus

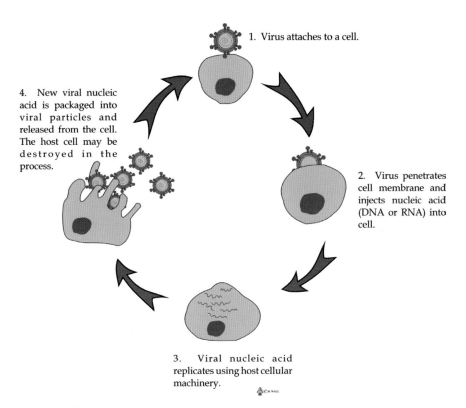

1. Virus attaches to a cell.

4. New viral nucleic acid is packaged into viral particles and released from the cell. The host cell may be destroyed in the process.

2. Virus penetrates cell membrane and injects nucleic acid (DNA or RNA) into cell.

3. Viral nucleic acid replicates using host cellular machinery.

The cycle of a virus.

the host cell's chemical machinery. As with dysbiosis and diseases, it isn't clear whether viruses come before dysbiosis or dysbiosis precedes viruses. We need more knowledge in this area before we can be certain, but early indications are that in many cases of ill health dysbiosis, viruses, autoimmunity and food sensitivities are all present in the same individual. It seems unlikely, according to the evidence available to us, that this is a coincidence.

Symptoms of viral infection:
1) Sexually transmitted diseases
2) Gastroenteritis
3) Pancreatitis

Symptoms of viral infection:
4) Skin infections
5) Cold/flus/pneumonia
6) Eye infections

Bacteria

Bacteria are single-celled organisms that grow almost ubiquitously on Earth. They are present in the environment, in the soil and in water. They are also found in plants and animals, including humans. We all have various species of bacteria living inside our intestinal tract and on our skin. While there are many beneficial species of bacteria, others are pathogenic and can cause illness. We generally think of being 'infected' by a bacteria from an outside source, but it is possible for some of the species that live inside of us, that are usually harmless, to overgrow and cause problems. Antibiotics and some other medications, as well as poor diet and lifestyle choices, can encourage this type of bacterial overgrowth.

Causes of bacterial overgrowth or bacterial infection:
1) Airborne bacterial contact
2) Skin contact
3) Water & food contamination
4) Antibiotics and acid-blocker medications (proton-pump inhibitors)
5) Sexual partner (exchange of saliva is enough to pass infection)
6) Pets

Symptoms of bacterial overgrowth or infection:
1) Skin infections
2) Abdominal pain, nausea, vomiting, constipation and diarrhoea
3) GERD
4) Respiratory symptoms (rhinitis/sinusitis, sore throat, pneumonia, cough, etc.)
5) Burning, pain with urination
6) Vaginal infections
7) Gingivitis
8) Fatigue

In summary, when dysbiosis is present, pathogens can find the host environment of dysbiotic humans an ideal place to set up home. Food and lifestyle choices can precipitate the creation of a perfect host environment for unwanted visitors. Once the bacterial environment and balance has changed in favour of parasites, viruses, pathogenic bacteria, yeast or fungal overgrowth they can dictate, to a degree, what foods we 'choose' to consume. All of these unwanted guests require energy and the simplest form of energy to guarantee their survival is sugar so people with dysbiosis tend to crave refined carbohydrates and sugars. We already know that poor dietary choices contribute to poor balance of gut bacteria. You can see how established dysbiosis could exacerbate the problem and lead us into a downward spiral.

Chapter 8

Stool Consistency and Gut Bacteria

The shape, size and colour of your stool as well as whether it floats or sinks can tell you an awful lot about your overall health and the balance of bacteria in your gut[71]. The appearance of stools and in particular, the colour and consistency, can even provide an indication of serious ill health or disease. The way a stool looks, smells and behaves in the toilet bowl provides a lot of useful clues too.

A healthy stool

A healthy stool should exit the body effortlessly, without pain and without the need to strain. It should be the tubular shape of a healthy colon, that is, the shape of a banana or a sausage. Of course there will be some smell but it shouldn't be foul or putrid. The stool will be moist and bulky and should slip out in one continuous solid log. Ideally, it will also be brown in colour. The normal colour of stools is a shade of brown. Any other colour, such as red, yellow, grey, white or green is not normal but could be due to colours of food eaten. Colour can indicate an unhealthy stool however, and should therefore be investigated to find out if there is a more serious cause.

Loosely formed stools

These stools may break off half way out of the back passage and stick a little, which can cause itching at the exit of the back passage as well as creating the feeling of incomplete emptying of the bowel. Straining is often required to dislodge this type of stool for complete evacuation. This type of stool is made when there is a lack of large amounts of bacteria and mucus. These normally combine to bond the contents of the stool together like glue. Bacterial mass can be increased by including soluble fibre and resistant starch in the diet, like cracked linseeds (soluble fibre) or an under ripe/green banana (resistant starch). Mucus tends to be present in a healthy, well digesting gut so optimising digestion is key to improving mucus production.

Watery, liquid stools

Watery stools are produced when too much water remains in the stool mass. This may be due to the inability of the colon to reabsorb the water because it did not remain in contact with the colon wall for long enough (it's moved through the body too quickly) or due to the release of water into the colon generally from toxins in the gut. Excessive amounts of some types of soluble fibre can cause fluid to be retained in the faecal mass and cause loose, soft stools.

Soluble fibre is important for the formation of the perfectly formed stool; however, it needs to be consumed with non-digestible insoluble fibre and resistant starch so that a solid stool is made. Insoluble fibre is found in the seeds and skins of fruit and vegetables, nuts, seeds as well as wholegrains. Resistant starch is a type of starch that isn't fully broken down and absorbed, but rather turned into short-chain fatty acids by intestinal bacteria. To get the most from resistant starch, choose whole, unprocessed sources of carbohydrate such as whole grains, fruits, vegetables, beans, legumes, cold cooked potatoes and rice as well as green (unripe) bananas.

Diarrhoea

Diarrhoea can have multiple causes:

1. Toxins secreted by microbes (bacteria and viruses).
2. Infections due to viruses, bacteria and parasites. These can affect the normal absorption and secretion processes of the gastrointestinal tract and cause retention of excessive amounts of water and electrolytes in the gut.
3. Inflammatory disease of the bowel (ulcerative colitis and Crohn's disease)
4. Malabsorption syndromes - lactose intolerance, coeliac disease (gluten intolerance) causes retention of water in the gut.

When diarrhoea strikes it's important to stay hydrated. That means consuming enough liquid to ensure you are excreting light yellow or straw-coloured urine. You may also need to replace some of your lost electrolytes (sodium and potassium) so coconut water and clear broths may help your recovery.

Pencil thin stools

Pencil thin stools may indicate an obstruction in the colon. Obstruction may be due to a mass in the colon that creates a blockage. When faeces are forced past this blockage, they tend be thinner and acquire a pencil thin shape. Inflammation, ulceration, polyps in the colon, a tumour or growth can lead to this type of stool. Many people produce this shaped stool from time to time but if you are doing so on a consistent basis you should visit your doctor for investigation so that any sinister causes can be eliminated.

Pale or grey coloured stool

The reason a healthy stool is brown is due to the bile acids which are produced by the bacterial breakdown of bile. A pale, grey or clay coloured stool indicates that there is too little bile being produced. The liver makes bile which is then stored in the gall bladder. It is squirted into the small intestine in response to the presence of fats. Bile salts emulsify the fats into smaller particles that can be broken down further by enzymes (Lipases) into fatty acids that may be absorbed through the intestinal wall. A lack of bile may be due to a slow production in the liver or a blockage of the tubes through which bile travels from the liver to the gall bladder and from the gall bladder into the intestines. Both of these possible causes need further investigation by your doctor.

Fatty stools

Fat is found in the stool when it escapes digestion and absorption in the small intestine, meaning it is still present when the stool is eliminated. This indicates a lack of digestive enzymes which are normally produced and secreted by the pancreas into the small intestines. This could be due to pancreatic insufficiency which is linked to other forms of ill health such as coeliac disease. We might all experience fatty stools from time to time. It is worth having a little look in the toilet bowl to check. However, if this happens a lot consider increasing your digestive enzyme secretion through better dietary choices or supplementation.

Pellet like stools or little lumps

Small lumps indicate that the stool has remained in the colon for too long, removing the water from the faeces. Slow gut transit causes retention of stool and continuous removal of water by the colon .The cause may be a lack of bulk in the diet. Insoluble fibre holds on to fluid and provides bulk to the stool. When the stool has no bulk, it cannot distend or stretch the muscular wall of the rectum and the reflex involved in making us want to pass a stool is not created. This type of stool is difficult to pass and often causes constipation. Diets that contain too much food from animal sources and very little from plant sources can contribute to this problem.

Dry or rock hard stools

These kinds of stools can also be produced by the removal of too much water from the faecal mass. The dried out stool is also difficult to pass, causing constipation. However, this problem may be due to slower gut function, not drinking enough fluids and not including enough fibre in the diet. Certain medications, including blood pressure drugs, anti-histamines, anti-depressants and painkillers like codeine, affect the speed of gut function and tend to slow down the movement of content down the tube.

Mucus in stools

Mucus in faeces comes from the lining of the gastrointestinal tract. Whilst we all produce some, too much mucus may indicate inflammation of the lining of the colon and rectum. This may be due to infections, perhaps from parasites or inflammatory bowel disease. Blood may also be present in these circumstances. This type of stool may adhere to the inside lining of the colon, rectum and anus and stimulate the urge to open the bowel repeatedly and lead to straining. Excessive gas may also be produced and occasionally this can result in accidental incontinence and soiling due to leakage.

Black, tarry, foul smelling stools

The black colour of a stool can indicate the presence of blood. The darker the stool, the higher up the digestive tract, the bleeding has stemmed from. Bloody stools are often a sign of an injury in the digestive tract. The term 'melena' is often used to describe black, tarry, and foul smelling stools. Certain medications that contain iron or bismuth may also produce black stools. This type of stool requires investigation and should be reported to your doctor without delay.

Bright red or bloody stools

Certain foods such as beetroot and tomatoes cause stools to be reddish but the major cause is due to the presence of blood. A streak of red in the stool together with red on the toilet tissue or toilet bowl is obviously blood and means bleeding along the gastrointestinal tract.

Fresh blood normally suggests blood from haemorrhoids or anal fissure but should be reported to your doctor if it persists so that other possible causes can be investigated. Slightly darker blood may suggest intestinal bleeding which could be due to ulcers, tumours, the bleeding associated with Crohn's disease, ulcerative colitis or perhaps even diverticulitis. Of course, this must also be reported to your doctor immediately.

Floating stool

A normal, healthy stool should sink to the bottom of the toilet bowl. However, stools often contain a large amount of gas as a result of bacterial fermentation and may float on top of the water in the toilet. While this doesn't indicate any specific disease, it can provide clues to dysbiosis and a presence of unwanted bacteria or yeast. Another reason that stools float is due to the presence of fat in the stool. This may indicate malabsorption of fat in the intestines as is the case with coeliac disease, however, this type of floating stool can be distinguished from others by the pale yellow colour and greasy texture with a foul smell.

This chart should help show the discrepancies between a healthy stool and an unhealthy stool.

	Healthy Stool	**Unhealthy Stool**
Colour:	Medium to light brown	Black, tarry or bright red stools may indicate bleeding in the GI tract; black stools can also come from certain medications and supplements (iron) White, pale or grey stools may indicate a lack of bile, which may suggest a serious problem (hepatitis, cirrhosis, pancreatic disorders, or possibly a blocked bile duct).
Consistency:	Smooth and soft, formed into one long shape and not a bunch of pieces	Hard lumps and pieces, or mushy and watery, or even pasty and difficult to clean off
Size and Shape:	About one to two inches in diameter and up to 18 inches long S-shaped, which reflects the shape of your lower intestine	Narrow, pencil-like or ribbon-like stools.
Texture:	Uniform texture	Presence of undigested food (more of a concern if accompanied by diarrhoea, weight loss, or other changes in bowel habits) Mucus in the stool. Floating stools can be a sign of food sensitivity or poor fat absorption.
Ease of passing:	Slip out easily without straining.	Stool that is hard to pass, painful, or requires straining

In summary, the way our stools look, smell and behave is a 'window' into the state of our gut health. It is one of many clues that may help us understand what is wrong with our digestion and how it may need treating. Bacterial imbalances can be the cause of suboptimal stools and these imbalances will need to be addressed before stools return to normal. One of the tools at our disposal for improving digestion and stool health is the addition of probiotics to our diet, either in the form of foods, supplements or both.

Chapter 9

What could probiotics do for me?

It is never too early to start thinking about probiotics and gut health. In fact, giving a baby regular doses through the mother's diet while it is still in the womb, and further along the line, through breastfeeding, may help to prevent health problems later in life. A study in 2008 [72] highlighted the potential for probiotic supplementation by mothers to boost the immune systems of infants. This is highly significant, especially in relation to children born via C-section, as it suggests that although these babies are at a disadvantage, for not having been born via the probiotic-rich birthing canal, they can in some ways make up for that through breastfeeding. Another positive outcome of early probiotic supplementation was shown in a 2012 study[73], which suggested that adding probiotics to mothers' diets during pregnancy and breastfeeding could reduce the risk of eczema in their offspring.

Studies suggest that using probiotics in the early years may well have an impact in later life. For some time, we have known that antioxidants play a key role in reducing the rate of ageing, while free radicals are responsible for speeding up the ageing process. The way to think about antioxidants and free radicals is like Pac-Man and the little pac-dots. Pac-Man (fuelled by antioxidants) travels through the maze (the bloodstream) to eat up the pac-dots (free radicals). Pac-Man has to stay fit, strong and healthy in order to eat up the pac-dots. Too many pac-dots left at the end of the game and you lose, or rather your health is diminished and you age more quickly. Studies show that probiotics may also act like antioxidants[74]. So by consuming and supplementing probiotics you makes your Pac-Man even stronger and better at its job of preventing illness and slowing down the ageing process.

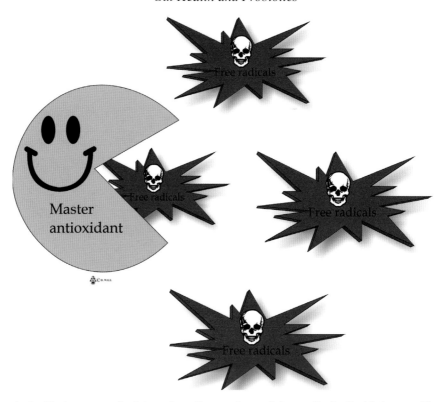

Antioxidants are required to reduce the numbers of free radicals. Probiotics act like antioxidants.

How do probiotics work?

There are four main ways in which probiotics work:

A. **Competition for nutrients.** By competing for available nutrients in the gastrointestinal tract, beneficial bacteria can inhibit the growth of other, less favourable bacteria.

B. **Blocking adhesion sites**. The addition of probiotics may actually stop pathogens from sticking to the cells of the gut. One study showed that L.acidophilus reduces the rate at which pathogens stick to human gut cells[75]. A similar and related way in which probiotics can work is by changing a toxin receptor, making the pathogen less harmful. Studies using Saccharomyces boulardii, a beneficial yeast, have shown positive results in making C. difficile (the virulent hospital bug) less harmful. [76]

C. **Immune stimulation**. This more systemic (bodywide) effect has been shown to help the immune system fight off pathogens. In one study, L. Rhamnosus (LGG) was given to Crohn's patients. The results showed

How Probiotics work

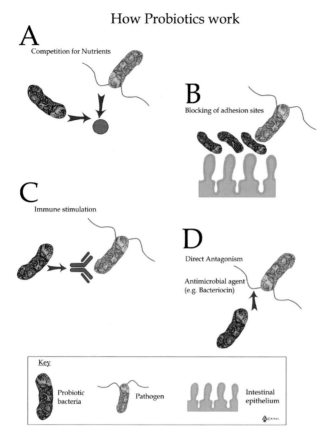

that the probiotic had beneficial effects on various markers of immune response and improved the patient's overall wellbeing. [77]

D. **Direct antagonism**. Probiotics may produce various antimicrobial substances. For instance, LGG produces substances that inhibit the spread of pathogens[78]. Other probiotics have also demonstrated direct antimicrobial activity as well. [79]

Probiotics to recover from ill health

There are many who believe that a malfunctioning digestive system is at the root of most illnesses. There's now a significant amount of research suggesting that an imbalance of beneficial-to-pathogenic bacteria and yeasts (dysbiosis) can disrupt the lining of the gut, whose role it is to defend the body against invading pathogens. So it seems that those who have encountered ill health may recover not by treating the symptoms but by treating the root cause of the illness i.e. the digestive system. Probiotics have been shown to play a crucial part in this recovery.

Lactose digestion

Lactose intolerance (LI), also known as lactose malabsorption, is the most common type of carbohydrate malabsorption. Lactose, of course, is the sugar found in milk. Intolerance to lactose exists due to low levels of lactase enzyme activity which means that lactose cannot be digested into its component parts. This results in bloating, cramping, flatulence and loose stools as unabsorbed lactose is broken down by colonic bacteria to produce gas. Symptoms tend to occur between thirty minutes to two hours after consumption.

Most people start life with a reasonable amount of the enzyme lactase so they are able to break down the lactose in milk. However, once weaned, many lose the ability to digest lactose as enzyme levels fall, and about sixty-five per cent of the world's population struggle to absorb lactose after infancy, The highest rates of LI (between sixty and a hundred per cent) are found in Asian populations, Native Americans and African Americans, while the lowest rates are found in people of northern European origin, including Northern Americans.

Studies have shown that people with lactose intolerance tolerate the lactose in yogurt better than the lactose in milk. Yogurt contains bacteria that actually produce the enzyme lactase. The presence of lactase producing bacteria in the yogurt, especially L. acidophilus, L. bulgaricus and S. thermophilus contribute to the digestion and absorption of lactose. The mechanism by which yogurt is better tolerated than milk by lactose intolerant individuals tell us that probiotics could help those with L.I. by increasing the levels of lactase present to break down the lactose in milk products.

Diarrhoea

Probiotics are useful in preventing and shortening the duration of several types of diarrhoea. A number of studies have noted that fermented milk products effectively prevent or treat infantile diarrhoea. Positive outcomes have been noted with L. casei and B. bifidum in particular. Other studies show that lactic acid bacteria can reduce the incidence of antibiotic-related diarrhoea.[80] This suggests a role for lactic acid bacteria in the treatment plan for people who routinely use antibiotics. Furthermore, studies have demonstrated the effectiveness of probiotics in decreasing the incidence of travellers' diarrhoea.[81] Whilst a lot of probiotic supplements have appeared on the market many people still travel without probiotics, especially to parts of the world renowned for leaving travellers with more than their luggage to transport back home. If gut bacteria are out of balance and opportunistic parasites or pathogenic bacteria are present, perhaps in food prepared by those with poor hygiene standards, you could end up with something in your gut that makes you feel very sick whilst you're away.

Effects on the immune system

The beneficial effects on the immune system are varied. Firstly, probiotics have been shown to enhance immune system function not just at the intestinal level but also at the systemic (whole body) level. They do this by increasing the levels of B-lymphocytes, whose job it is to recognise and destroy foreign invaders, by boosting levels of IgA-, IgG- and IgM-secreting cells and serum IgA levels, all of which increase the antibody activity of the body.

It has also been proven that probiotic bacteria can stimulate the activity of the intestinal mucosa. The mucosa provides a physical barrier that prevents foreign substances from passing through the gut. Lots of immune cells are found in the gut mucosa. These cells allow the gut to interact with the immune system. It is believed that this is the mechanism by which the probiotic Lactobacillus GG has been shown to reverse leaky i.e. by increasing the activity of the gut mucosa thereby strengthening the lining of the gut[82].

Probiotic bacteria can also play a role in treating food allergy. This was demonstrated in an experiment with infants known to have eczema due to a cow's milk allergy[83]. Infants in the experimental group were given hydrolysed whey formula fortified with LGG, whilst those in the control group just got whey formula. The skin condition of the infants getting the LGG improved significantly compared to the control group. In addition, the experimental group saw a reduction of inflammation of the intestine.

In fact, there are a number of health issues that have shown improvements after the administration of certain probiotics:

Health Issue	Probiotics
Acne	L. rhamnosus SP1
Antibiotic related diarrhoea	L. acidophilus and L.rhamnosus [84] Saccharomyces boulardii
Candida	L. rhamnosus[85], L. acidophilus and L. reuteri RC-14
Cholesterol	L. plantarum, L. reuteri
Constipation	B. lactis BB-12[86, 87]
Eczema	L. rhamnosus HN001, L. Fermentum VRI-003 PCC
Colds and Flue	B. animalis lactis Bi-07 and L. acidophilus NCFM
Halitosis (bad breath), periodontitis, gingivitis	L. reuteri LR-1 or LR-2
H. Pylori	L. johnsonii
IBS	B. bifidum MIMBb75, B. infantis 35624, and L. plantarum 299V

Health Issue	Probiotics
Lactose Intolerance	L. acidophilus, L. bulgaricus, and Streptococcus thermophiles
Food Poisoning	L. murinus and one strain each of L. salivarius subsp. salivarius, L. pentosus, and Pediococcus pentosaceous
Travellers' Diarrhoea	L. acidophilus, B. bifidum, Saccharomyces boulardii [88]

How to choose a probiotic supplement?

In order to choose the right probiotic for you, first consider that it must survive your stomach acid, bile and digestive enzymes so that it is still intact when and where in your digestive tract it is needed. Its role is to prevent pathogens and allergens from binding to cells in the gut, and it must also be able to fight off pathogenic bacteria, viruses, fungi and parasites. Finally, it must be safe and well-tolerated. That's quite a lot to ask from one little pill and as you can imagine, many of the cheaper products on the market might fall short of one or more of these demanding roles. So here are some pointers of what to look out for on the label:

- Be reassured that if your probiotic contains the most researched strains, lactobacillus and bifidobacteria, you are in the right area to begin with.
- Look for a probiotic that contains at least a few billion active bacteria. Whilst opinions vary, between 2 and 10 billion is reasonable. The label should also advise how many organisms are contained in a single dose and how often you should take it.
- It's helpful if the label tells you how many viable organisms there are in the product at its expiration date, since this will be less than when they are manufactured. This figure guarantees the minimum dose you will receive.
- The label on your probiotic should advise that the probiotics are resistant to stomach acid, or can be dissolved in water so that they pass through the stomach environment fairly quickly and reach the parts of the gastrointestinal tract where they are needed most OR make sure it is in an encapsulated pill form or other delayed-rupture technology so they reach their destination.
- Genus, species and strain of the microorganisms should be included on the label.
- Ensure the label specifies storage information when relevant. Some forms need to be refrigerated while others need a dark, cool space. Always keep probiotics away from moisture and heat.

A note of caution

There are a lot of probiotics that cannot survive the transportation and storage process. Probiotics are very delicate bacteria. The truth is that when the supplements leave the manufacturer, they have to be shipped on trucks, and sit on store shelves or in warehouses. Due to their transportation, the power of these bacteria will have diminished, or worse, completely disappeared by the time you purchase them. Furthermore, some probiotics are dead by the time they arrive in your intestines. In order to limit the possibility of purchasing probiotics that are dead or do not reach the site of action then do your research on the supplement you actually need or which combination you need to address your symptoms; be sure to look into the company you want to purchase the probiotic from as well as the information outlined above. If you're satisfied by the product itself, the manufacturer and the channel (shop either online or offline) then go ahead and make your purchase.

Contraindications

Probiotics are generally considered safe with bloating and flatulence being the most likely side effects. These side effects may mean you are not taking the right combination for your gut. You may need to experiment to get the right probiotic for you. Probiotics should be used cautiously in patients who are critically ill or severely immunocompromised. This is because systemic infections may occur, though they are extremely rare. Bacteria-derived probiotics should also be taken at least two hours before or after antibiotics.

How to take?

Probiotics should be taken in combinations, not alone as that's how probiotics appear in nature. Take your probiotic supplement with food or as instructed on the bottle for four weeks and make an assessment as to whether that combination has made a difference. If not, then you may need to look at a different combination. Remember to consider which probiotic strains have been shown to improve the health conditions that affect you.

Boosting probiotic levels without supplementation

It's also possible to boost your intake and uptake of probiotics by making a few tweaks to your current dietary plan.

- Sour and pickled foods like apple cider vinegar and fermented vegetables such as sauerkraut contain some probiotics, as well as certain types of acids that help to create the right pH balance in our gut to support and benefit the probiotics in our system.

- Probiotic foods such as naturally fermented yogurt (goat's yogurt tends still to be produced through natural fermentation and some of the better brands on the market will produce their cows milk yogurt this way too), kefir, kimchi, kombucha can all boost our probiotic levels.
- Prebiotic foods can help probiotics to thrive in our gut. These effectively feed the probiotics in our system. The soluble fibre which is also called fermentable fibre is found in vegetables, fruits and also in chia and flaxseeds.
- Resistant starch found in cold potatoes, rice and legumes but also in unripe bananas and plantains can also help probiotic bacteria to thrive

In summary, additional probiotics can be obtained from supplements or from the food we eat and the drinks we consume. They can be encouraged to work optimally for us by consuming foods and drinks that create the right environment and those that provide the fuel for probiotics to thrive. When choosing a supplement, it's important to do your research first, looking into the manufacturer and delivery method. Expect to pay for what you get in general. Consider supplementing with probiotics if you have symptoms related to dysbiosis or if you are due to take medication like NSAIDs or antibiotics, that will negatively impact gut bacteria.

Chapter 10

Probiotics and Antibiotics – are they opposing forces?

A question that people often ask, once they understand the preventative role of probiotics, is, 'Do I ever really need antibiotics?" The answer is an unequivocal YES but only in certain circumstances and this is where confusion is putting pressure on global healthcare systems. Probiotics also have a place in medicine but they are currently being underused and perhaps that's because their role is also misunderstood.

The vital role of antibiotics.

Antibiotics save lives. There is absolutely no doubt that they play a fundamental role in clearing up life-threatening bacterial infections. We know that antibiotics have saved millions of lives around the world since they began being used on humans.

Antibiotics were originally discovered by Alexander Fleming back in 1928. What Fleming discovered gives the vital clue as to when and how antibiotics should be used in practice. While he was clearing up his laboratory, he was tidying away some petri dishes that had staphylococcus bacteria on them. He noticed that where mould had been allowed to build up on some of the plates, the staphylococcus bacteria had been killed off. This mould was called penicillin notatum. When, ten years later, a couple of scientists at Oxford University managed to isolate the bacteria killing penicillin, the practical use of antibiotics was realised. It was subsequently mass produced by an American pharmaceutical company which meant there was enough to save many lives during the Second World War. When antibiotics are appropriately prescribed they play an essential role in saving lives, something that cannot be stressed enough.

Antibiotic Prescriptions – Too Much Too Often

What is of concern, however, is the frequency with which antibiotics are now prescribed and the quantities that are prescribed without proper assessment of their effectiveness. Too often, antibiotics are prescribed where they are not actually necessary. They are, for instance, ineffective in the treatment of viral infections. By their very nature, antibiotics target bacteria. Sadly, for various different reasons, doctors prescribe antibiotics when the likelihood of them being effective is very low.

Furthermore, there is an argument that many bacterial infections could be cleared by the body's own immune system if it is given the chance to step up. In this way, the body builds up resistance to a repeat infection, and it automatically fights off food poisoning and certain skin infections without antibiotic intervention. For this reason, doctors will sometimes prescribe antibiotics to a patient but ask that they do not complete the prescription unless they absolutely need to. Doctors know that the infection may well clear up all by itself but they won't have the time to see the patient again in a couple of days. This method of 'delayed prescribing' means you can often save your body from unnecessary exposure to antibiotics. Ideally, this practice would be used more often, and patients would be made aware of the issues of over prescription. Sadly, we have now reached a state of antibiotic resistance which is proving to be another threat to life.

Antibiotic resistance

Overuse and misuse of antibiotics has led to a rise in antibiotic resistance. Antibiotic resistance occurs when bacteria are no longer sensitive to a medication that should eliminate an infection. Antibiotic-resistant bacterial infections are potentially very dangerous and increase the risk of death. In the UK alone, the consumption of systemic antibiotics and intestinal antibiotics in humans equated to 135mg per kg of human biomass in 2013[89] . Some would argue that this exceeds our need for antibiotics and it is this level of consumption that has led to the current situation where many infections are simply resistant to antibiotics and therefore untreatable.

An estimated 25,000 people die each year in the European Union from antibiotic-resistant bacterial infections. One of the infections causing the most deaths due to antibiotic-resistance is Clostridium difficile (C. difficile). This is a common infection transmitted, ironically, in hospitals and nursing homes.

The issue of antibiotic-resistance is not going away and is getting worse. Now, governments and even the World Health Organisation (WHO) are stepping in to try and halt the problem. While some of the onus is on the medical and healthcare professions to prescribe antibiotics ONLY when needed, patients also need to be aware that some infections are better off left to take their natural course.

How Antibiotic Resistance Occurs

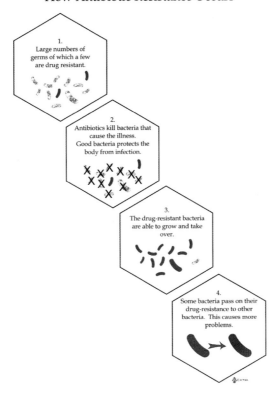

1.
Large numbers of germs of which a few are drug resistant.

2.
Antibiotics kill bacteria that cause the illness.
Good bacteria protects the body from infection.

3.
The drug-resistant bacteria are able to grow and take over.

4.
Some bacteria pass on their drug-resistance to other bacteria. This causes more problems.

Can you replace antibiotics with probiotics?

In the face of so many issues with antibiotic over prescription and misuse you might think that the solution lies in probiotics. Well, while antibiotics kill off both the disease causing bacteria and the healthy bacteria too, there's still a case for using them when necessary. However, there are also infections that could and have been cleared by treating more naturally, through probiotics and lifestyle changes, and one such example is the treatment of acne. Skin conditions such as acne have a history of being treated using antibiotics. Yet, several studies have reported beneficial effects for acne sufferers following the use of probiotics combined with some changes to diet. In an article by the American Academy of Dermatology[90] expert Dr Witney Bowe explained that oral probiotics could influence skin conditions such as acne and rosacea by affecting what is known as the 'gut-brain-skin axis.'

As the digestive system becomes slow and sluggish so the bacterial balance in the gut can change, allowing gaps to form between the epithelial cells of the gut (also known as 'Leaky Gut Syndrome'). These gaps in the lining of the gut allow toxins to be released into the bloodstream and this causes an inflammatory

Potential pathways of the Gut-Brain-Skin axis in acne vulgaris

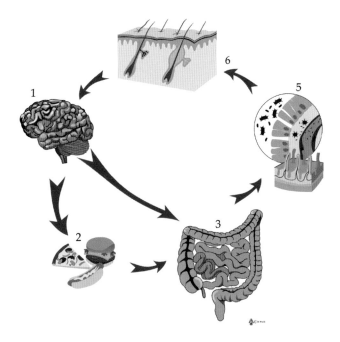

response by the body's immune system. If there is a genetic predisposition to acne then an individual can experience a flare-up as a result of this change to their gut bacteria and the resulting inflammation.

Based on the path to this state of imbalance, the way to address poor skin health is to reverse the causes. Firstly, find ways to reduce exposure to stress and in particular, make changes to diet. Importantly, the introduction of healthy bacteria to the gut in the form of probiotics can help greatly. The probiotics will help to boost the population of immune boosting 'good' bacteria in the gut. This, in turn, will help improve the overall gut health and give it a chance to heal and seal, creating an impermeable barrier that prevents inflammation that can trigger acne. This is an area of increasing interest, and there are some studies of note that outline how probiotics could be used in place of antibiotics in the treatment of acne.

In one twelve week Korean study[91] a fermented milk drink, rich in probiotics, proved to significantly decrease acne in terms of reducing the number of acne lesions and the acne grade as well as reducing the amount of surface oil, compared to the placebo. No alterations in skin hydration or pH occurred in either group. In an Italian study[92], supplementation with lactobacillus rhamnosus SP1 also improved the appearance of adult acne.

Furthermore, in a review of the data[93] on the use of probiotics for acute diarrhoea in children, in two studies, it was found that probiotics shorten the duration of diarrhoea and reduce the stool frequency on day five. In a third study, (of four in total reviewed) it was found that probiotics reduce the hospital stay period.

So there are some examples of bacterial infections which can be improved using probiotics without antibiotic intervention.

Taking probiotics alongside antibiotics

We have discovered that antibiotics have a really important role to play in killing off pathogenic bacteria, but they also destroy good gut bacteria too, and as a result of this, some people will suffer from antibiotic induced diarrhoea, constipation or even an overgrowth of unwanted yeast. The most common of these side effects is diarrhoea. In fact, it is so common that it has its own acronym, ADD (antibiotic associated diarrhoea). There have been many studies carried out to find out if taking probiotics at the same time as antibiotics might help reduce this unwanted side effect. The good news is that research shows that probiotics do have a positive effect and do reduce the risk of diarrhoea. A 2016 study[94] concluded that supplementation with specific probiotics, namely L. helveticus and L. rhamnosus significantly reduced the duration of diarrhoea in healthy adults receiving antibiotics. This study and others have shown that probiotics can be effective in preventing or reducing the severity of ADD in those taking antibiotics.

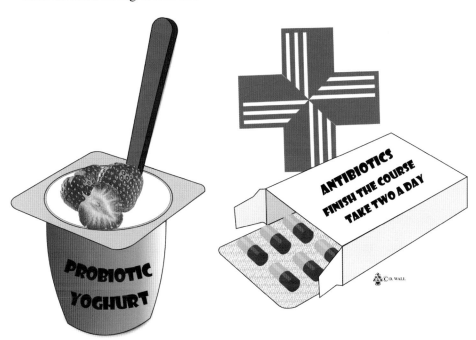

There are also conclusive studies on the administration of probiotics alongside antibiotics in the treatment of bacterial vaginosis. One such study[95] enrolled 125 premenopausal women with diagnosed bacterial infections of the vagina. Eighteen women were given the standard antibiotic therapy, consisting of metronidazole (500 mg), taken twice a day for one week. Additionally, subjects were randomly assigned to take a dose of oral probiotics twice a day, containing L. rhamnosus GR-1 and L. reuteri RC-14, or a placebo dose, for a month, starting on the first day of treatment with the antibiotic. At the end of the trial, eighty-eight per cent of women taking both antibiotic and oral probiotics were judged to have been cured by their treatment. In complete contrast to this phenomenal rate, only forty per cent of the women taking standard antibiotics on their own were judged to have been cured. In addition, the lactobacillus counts were high in ninety-six per cent of the women who had received probiotic therapy, while counts were high in only fifty-three per cent of control subjects (i.e. those who had taken the placebo) at the end of the study.

Taking probiotics and antibiotics together is therefore a good option for a bacterial infection that couldn't be cured by leaving it to your body's own immune system. However, the timing of the probiotics and antibiotics dosages is crucial to the effectiveness of both. According to probiotic expert, Dr Nigel Plummer PhD[96] we should never take probiotics and antibiotics at exactly the same time. They should never be in the stomach together. The ideal situation is, if the antibiotic is being taken at the start and end of the day then the probiotic should be taken at lunchtime. If that is not possible then the probiotic must be taken at least two hours before or after the antibiotic in order to get the beneficial effects of both.

When it comes to choosing probiotics instead of antibiotics, it is fair to say that we are still in a situation where if antibiotics have been prescribed and you're already taking them, then you must carry on taking them. Many people stop taking their antibiotic before the course has finished. This is sometimes due to unwanted side effects and sometimes due to the patient feeling better or simply forgetting to take their pills regularly. The reason this is not a good idea is that at the beginning of treatment antibiotics wipe out the most vulnerable and weakest bacteria. If you stop the course early, you'll allow relatively resistant bacteria to survive and multiply. Not only do they survive, but since they have been 'spotted' by the antibiotics, they can change their structure so that antibiotics will not be actively able to wipe them out in the future.

Don't stop consuming probiotics the moment your course of antibiotics is complete

AAD (antibiotic associated diarrhoea) can start several weeks after completing a course of antibiotics. Your gut changes a lot whilst you are taking antibiotics and in the period afterwards. This change can happen over a period of months as your body adjusts both to the infection that caused you to have to take the antibiotics in the first place and then the antibiotics themselves. Therefore, probiotic supplementation is likely to have a benefit for weeks after completing a course of antibiotics, particularly in terms of boosting your natural population of friendly bacteria. Once you're clear of the risk of AAD, it is still recommended that you introduce your post-infection gut to a wide variety of beneficial bugs. These can come from consuming fermented foods rich in probiotics like kefir, kombucha, sauerkraut, kimchi, miso soup and tempeh, as well as from dietary supplements if required.

So, in summary, the future for probiotics looks bright. There's more and more proof that they are effective in treating infectious diseases. There's also evidence suggesting that they can provide a useful addition to antibiotic treatment in some cases, too. As increasing evidence emerges of their role both alone and alongside antibiotics, we have a clearer picture of what probiotic species are best for which illness and which species complement specific antibiotics in the treatment and prevention of infectious diseases. At a point in the future, we may well be able to raise the question of probiotics vs antibiotics, and which ones doctors ought to prescribe. For now, however, certainly where serious health conditions are concerned, it simply isn't a question of probiotics OR antibiotics - it's a matter of probiotics AND antibiotics. We are starting to see just how effective probiotic intervention can be for less serious health conditions and the results are very promising indeed.

Chapter 11

Leaky Gut Syndrome and Food Sensitivities

'Leaky Gut' is used to describe something called intestinal permeability, and it is a term that makes some medical professionals feel uncomfortable, possibly because it doesn't sound very medically sophisticated, and also as it is now linked to so many different illnesses that it seems insufficient for such an all-encompassing condition. Regardless of its name, the fact is that more and more people are suffering from it.

Why the gut should not be leaky

A huge proportion of our immune system sits within the tissues that surround the gut. You can think of your gut as the inner tube of a bike tyre. It's the essential barrier between the world outside and the inside. Although there are several compartments to the long tube that is called our digestive tract, partially digested food particles should never actually be able to leak out into the main body of a person, neither should bacteria either 'good' or 'bad'. When they do, it spells trouble.

Absorption of nutrients is a multifactorial process. Food has to be broken down into its simplest form in order to be absorbed from the small intestine into the body. It does this with a combination of acid and enzymes that are produced by the cells that line the stomach, and some bile salts made by the liver, but stored and released from the gall bladder and also, importantly, the gut bacteria. In order to be efficiently absorbed each food group has to be broken down into a simpler form of its former self:

Ingested Form	Simplest Component
Carbohydrates	Monosaccharides (simple sugars)
Fat	Fatty Acids
Protein	Amino Acids

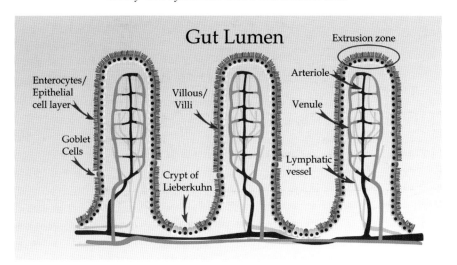

These simpler components are then transported into the body from the gut. The 'postmen' here are called 'enterocytes'. It's the enterocytes' job to make sure that simple sugars, fatty acids and amino acids get transported from the gut side of cells to the body side of cells.

Once they're on the other side of the gut, cells, amino acids and sugars are transported in the blood alongside minerals and water-soluble vitamins. Meanwhile, fatty acids and fat soluble vitamins are transported in lymph vessels by the lymphatic system.

Mucus is secreted by cells on the perimeter of the gut. This mucus forms a layer which becomes a physical barrier between the gut and the body. On the gut side of each enterocyte are finger-like projections called microvilli. They are finger-like in order to maximise the nutrients available for nutrient absorption.

When does leaky gut occur?

Now imagine that the inner tube belongs to a bike that has been left to rust in the garage for some time. The balding outside layer of the inner tube has started to split a little at the edges, it looks like an arid, parched landscape on the outside but it's still just about doing its job of holding the air in and keeping debris out. Then you decide to take the bike for a ride, and as you hit a bump, some debris in the road penetrates the tyre. This debris can be thought of as inflammation. Once it is allowed into the inner tube (digestive tract), more and more debris is able to enter. Then the already parched surface of the inner tube starts to break up. What was once on the inside of the inner tube is now able to leak through the inner tube and into the tyre itself. That's akin to the particles of food that should be broken down by the small intestine leaking out into the body.

What is waiting on the other side of the gut are our immune cells. They recognise the 'leaked particles' as foreign invaders and launch an immune attack against them. When large quantities of particles have escaped, other parts of the immune system are fired up to help the immune response. The lymph system and liver both get involved at this stage, and it is this body-wide effect that can lead to systemic inflammation.

When pathogenic substances such as bacteria or even toxins leak out of the gut and into the body the resulting cytokine release (the chemical messengers that communicate with other cells in the body) cause generalised inflammation without a specific target. This may explain why some people experience joint pain as a result of intestinal permeability and others might experience brain fog for example.

When incompletely digested proteins stimulate the immune system, it's the adaptive (acquired) immune system that gets involved. That is the part of the immune system that remembers the initial response to a pathogen, or in this case an undigested protein, and makes subsequent reactions worse every time

Inside the gut

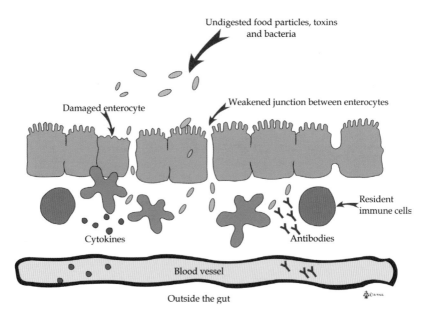

The immune system reacts when it finds undigested proteins where they shouldn't normally be in a healthy body.

72

the body is exposed to that pathogen or protein. This may be why allergies form. Allergies occur when cells secrete Immunoglobulin E (IgE) antibodies that target a part of a protein that is specific to a food, such as milk or peanuts. It's the protein in milk called casein that causes milk allergy and the allergens in peanuts have been identified as proteins called Ara h 1, Ara h 2, and Ara h 3. If these are incompletely digested, then the immune system will launch an attack, and each subsequent attack will be more dramatic.

The liver is also put under strain by this invasion from the digestive tract. Its role is to break down the substances that have leaked out of the gut. Its ability to achieve this depends on how much work it is already doing. If the liver is already coping with medication, hormone imbalances and stress, for example, this toxic load may simply push it over the limit. The liver is the gut's close ally and without it operating fully, we can enter a downward spiral as health declines.

Health conditions linked to leaky gut

Not everyone with intestinal permeability will experience ill health. A handful of studies have shown that healthy relatives of people with autoimmune conditions can have intestinal permeability but be completely asymptomatic. How do they know they have leaky gut in the first place, you may ask. Well, they can be tested – more about this in the next chapter.

Also for some, there may be signs of intestinal permeability in the body without any gastrointestinal symptoms. For example, vitamin and mineral deficiencies or inflammation can show up. Unfortunately there are lots of health conditions linked to Leaky Gut Syndrome and amongst the most common is food sensitivity. What's more, is that increasingly, we are able to link autoimmune diseases and food sensitivities. The correlation between the two is no big surprise except perhaps to those millions of people worldwide who have no idea that what they are eating could be making their autoimmune symptoms far worse. Studies now link autoimmune diseases and leaky gut in a range of health issues:

Autoimmune Conditions linked with Leaky Gut:
Inflammatory Joint Disease[97]
Inflammatory Bowel Disease[98] [99]
Coeliac Disease[100]
Autoimmune Skin Conditions[101]
HIV[102]

Triggers for leaky gut

Whilst our body is designed to cope with a certain amount of stress, it doesn't respond so well to the volume and frequency of stress we face today. This kind of stress changes the body's immune system and results in it producing less secretory IgA (part of our immune system), less DHEA (an anti-stress hormone) and it also slows down the rate of digestion which means food hangs around in the intestinal tract for longer, producing more toxins that can then circulate in the body and cause havoc.

Dysbiosis is another trigger for leaky gut syndrome but some of the causative factors in dysbiosis may also be triggers for leaky gut; excess alcohol, poor dietary choices, medication, and even surgery can trigger leaky gut.

Food Allergy and Leaky Gut

The relationship between food sensitivities and leaky gut is complex and circular. Children and adults with eczema, urticaria (hives) or asthma triggered by atopic food allergy tend to have far more permeable guts than those without these conditions. Following exposure to allergenic foods, permeability sharply increases. This is due to the release of histamine which can cause inflammation in the body that in turn, accelerates the progress of intestinal permeability. There is a cause and effect relationship between atopic diseases and food allergies.

How the liver is affected by leaky gut

Herein lies another cycle. When leaky gut is present, the liver is put under more strain and has to work overtime to remove unwanted toxins. Toxins leak out of the gut and travel to the liver where they pile more of a load onto the liver. During this process, the liver produces a larger number of free radicals and so the antioxidant requirements of the body go up. Toxins also stimulate immune cells in the liver. This causes inflammation. Inflammation can cause further leaky gut issues and place even greater strain on the liver. As the antioxidant requirements go up so too does the need for probiotics.

Food intolerance

The truth of the matter is that food intolerance is a very real issue that is responsible for a whole host of health symptoms. When food and drink are digested, the proteins within them are broken down into smaller fragments for easy absorption into the body. When partially broken down food particles enter the body, it sometimes reacts by attacking those particles, using antibodies called Immunoglobulin G's (IgG).

A recent study[103] showed that those who eliminated trigger foods based on food-specific IgG test results had reductions in weight, body mass index, waist and hip circumference and improvements in all indicators of quality of life that were measured. These included physical and emotional wellbeing, mental health, social life, pain levels and vitality.

There's much confusion when it comes to the definition and differences between food intolerance and food allergy. But they are very different things, as we shall see below:

Food Intolerance	Food Allergy
Reactions up to 72 hours after eating	Immediate reactions (2 hours or less)
Multiple foods can be involved	Rarely more than 1 to 2 foods (although there are exceptions)
Any organ system can be affected	Primarily skin, airways and digestive system
Very common	Trace amounts of foods can cause reactions
Difficult to self-diagnose	Caused by raised IgE antibody
Symptoms can clear after avoidance for a period and following gut healing.	Lifelong (some people grow out of early childhood allergies)

Food intolerance is a condition with a wide range of symptoms, including stomach issues, bloating, migraines, low mood, weight gain, and fatigue and skin problems.

Symptoms of Food Intolerance			
Abdominal Pain	Dizziness	Hyperactivity	Tension
Aches and Pains	Eczema	Migraine	Tiredness
Acne	Fatigue	Nausea	Urticaria
Bloating	Irritable Bowel Syndrome (IBS)	Rashes	Weight loss/ Weight Gain
Constipation	Itching	Rhinitis	Wheezing
Chronic Fatigue Syndrome	Fluid Retention	Sinusitis	
Diarrhoea	Headaches	Stomach Cramps	

Symptoms of food intolerance can take up to seventy-two hours to appear after eating the trigger food or group of foods. On average, people who suffer from food intolerances usually have between four and eight trigger foods. Many people suffer for years, having formed a coping mechanism to deal with the symptoms but being unable to enjoy a normal work and home life. They don't realise that there are easy steps to take that could resolve their condition. A gut healing programme to address the underlying problem i.e. the leaky gut should help to address certain food intolerances too.

Fructose malabsorption

The number of people suffering with fructose intolerance is greatly underestimated due to poor diagnosis both on behalf of medical professionals and patients themselves. Incompletely absorbed (malabsorbed) fructose is fermented by the flora in the large intestine, resulting in the formation of gas and chemical substances, including short-chain fatty acids. The threshold of fructose malabsorption varies individually and widely. Most individuals will show malabsorption of sugars, including fructose, only when very large quantities are consumed.

Many people are diagnosed with this condition later in life. The reason is because the activity of the transport proteins facilitating gut absorption of fructose is altered by inflammation or stress. However, another reason for later diagnosis is that the microbiome can also change after intestinal infections or antibiotic use.

Fructose is found in honey, various fruits and often in sweetened snacks or drinks in daily amounts of at least 20 – 70g, depending on the local diet. Some sports and fruit drinks contain over 50g of fructose per 100ml which for anyone with fructose malabsorption would prove uncomfortable. Fructose consumption has increased markedly in the last decades due to the use of fructose as a sweetener in many processed foods, even savoury ones. Also we can now buy the sweetest of fruit, including pineapple, banana and mango, or even dried fruits, all year round unlike our ancestors who would have eaten fruit in small quantities and seasonally.

Fodmap Sensitivity

The acronym FODMAP refers to a collection of short chain carbohydrates and sugar alcohols found in food. Fructose is one of these carbohydrates but also included are fructans, galacto-oligosaccharides, lactose and polyols e.g. sorbitol and mannitol. These carbohydrates and sugar alcohols are readily fermented by bacteria in the large intestine which produces gas. They're also osmotic, meaning they attract water into large intestine which can alter how quickly and efficiency bowels move. People with FODMAP sensitivity tend to present with various IBS symptoms. It's almost impossible to avoid all foods containing FODMAPs so a low FODMAP diet is advised. However, the underlying cause for FODMAP sensitivity should also be investigated. See Chapter 22 for more information on FODMAP foods.

Lactose intolerance

Lactose intolerance (LI) is a condition that affects an estimated seventy-five per cent of people globally. Lactose is the sugar found in varying amounts in dairy products. In order to digest this sugar properly, the small intestine produces an enzyme called lactase. Lactase is responsible for breaking down the lactose into glucose and galactose, so the body can absorb it. When the body's ability to make lactase diminishes, the result is lactose intolerance. Then the body is exposed and reacts to the lactose still present. Yogurt and kefir (a fermented probiotic milk drink) both with live active cultures typically do not produce the symptoms, as the active cultures help to break down lactose prior to consumption.

Coeliac disease

Coeliac disease remains one of the most challenging illnesses associated with the small intestine. It involves multiple pathways and there is no medication available yet to cure it. Normal gut bacteria have a vital role in maintaining the intestinal balance and promoting health. Coeliac disease is associated with gut bacteria alteration, especially with an increase in the number of undesirable bacteria and a decrease in the number of probiotic bacteria. There is a strong relationship between intestinal dysbiosis and coeliac disease, and recent studies are aimed at determining whether coeliac disease is a risk factor for dysbiosis or dysbiosis is a risk factor for coeliac disease. Either way balancing gut bacteria is a suitable approach for anyone suffering from coeliac disease.

Non-coeliac gluten sensitivity

People with gluten sensitivity would not test positive for coeliac disease based on blood testing, nor do they have the same type of intestinal damage found in individuals with coeliac disease. However, they are still unable to tolerate gluten. In this disease, partially digested proteins (gliadin and gluten peptides) cause an inflammatory reaction once they have been identified by the immune system as foreign invaders. As a result, a chemical called zonulin is produced by the gut wall cells which are linked to increasing the permeability of the gut. Zonulin was identified by Dr Alessio Fasano in 2000. For this reason, even without a coeliac diagnosis, elimination of gluten and balancing gut bacteria would be suitable strategies for those suffering from gluten sensitivity.[104]

In summary, leaky gut or intestinal permeability is a key element in many different diseases. Permeability starts a process, a vicious cycle if you like, in which allergic sensitisation, immune activation, liver dysfunction, pancreatic insufficiency and malnutrition, occur. In turn, each of these conditions increases the leakiness of the small bowel. Effective treatment of leaky gut syndrome requires several components, including avoidance of allergic foods, elimination of infection or bacterial overgrowth with antimicrobials and probiotics, and dietary supplementation. Direct measurement of intestinal permeability can help identify appropriate strategies and to gauge the effectiveness of treatment. Certainly, dietary intervention combined with therapeutic care can reap rewards and help to start healing a leaky gut.

Chapter 12

Gut Tests

The importance of testing

One good reason to take a look at what's happening inside your gut is that there are links between the health of the gut microbiome and the development of serious health problems. Abnormalities in the gut microbiome have been reported in patients with colorectal cancer for example. Joseph P. Zackular and colleagues[105] looked at stool samples of three groups of people representing three stages of colorectal cancer. They found a correlation between the levels of specific bacteria and the presence of tumours. Yet microbiome screening is not yet used as a diagnostic tool for this disease.

Other illnesses, amongst them autoimmune diseases, such as MS, diabetes type 1 and coeliac disease, are also linked to changes or abnormalities in the microbiome. Perhaps screening should be considered as part of the diagnosis process for these illnesses. Indeed if stool testing could be used to detect the presence of precancerous and cancerous lesions or of an increased risk of MS, then perhaps preventative measures could be put in place, rectifying the microbiome abnormalities through intervention. Even if you do not suspect an autoimmune disease or a serious illness, you may feel that something is not right with your gut or your overall health and that the gut may be the root cause. This chapter explores the main tests available for identifying what underlying gut health issues need addressing in order to achieve better health.

Do you need to take a test?

To identify if you could benefit from a test on your digestive system, ask yourself the following questions:

- Do you suffer from IBS?
- Do you get indigestion?
- Do you suffer from either constipation or diarrhoea or both?
- Do you get stomach distention i.e. pain and bloating or just bloating?
- Are you more 'gassy' than you used to be?

- Have you been diagnosed with an inflammatory bowel condition such as Crohn's disease or ulcerative colitis?
- Do you suffer from unexplained fatigue?
- Have you been diagnosed with rheumatoid arthritis?
- Do you have food allergies or intolerance?
- Are you suffering from an autoimmune condition?
- Do you have a skin condition such as psoriasis, acne or eczema?
- Have you used antibiotics for a period of time in the past?

Answering yes to any of these questions means you could benefit from a digestive analysis test. Below we will have a look at some of the tests available:

Comprehensive Stool Analysis

Probably the most frequently used digestive test, this is a comprehensive assessment of someone's ability to digest and absorb nutrients. It is also used to check levels of 'good' and 'bad' bacteria, such as lactobacillus and bifidobacteria and yeasts like candida. It does not, however, include the detection of intestinal parasites. This test is normally useful to people with poor digestion and poor absorption. Most commonly, those with both are likely to be suffering from IBS symptoms, and constipation and/or diarrhoea and this test helps to identify the possible causes.

Comprehensive Stool Analysis with Parasitology

This test includes all of the elements of the comprehensive stool analysis but looks for intestinal parasites and parasite eggs as well. In addition to digestion and absorption issues, those with a parasitic infection may also suffer from skin itching (and hives) as well as anal itching, unexplained fever, possible weight loss or gain, aching muscles, nausea and fatigue.

What's involved in taking these tests?

This is a simple test that requires you to collect stool samples in your own home before transferring to a laboratory via courier. Samples are taken over three consecutive days.

Small Intestinal Bacterial Overgrowth (SIBO) Breath Test

SIBO is vastly underdiagnosed. This may be due to a lack of diagnostic knowledge on the part of medical professionals. However, SIBO may be present in anywhere from thirty to thirty-five per cent[106, 107] of IBS cases. It may also help explain why some coeliac sufferers are not responsive to a gluten free diet. SIBO was discovered in nearly ten per cent of those with coeliac disease who are not responding to a gluten-free diet[108]. SIBO could also be a factor in weight gain. One study performed on asymptomatic morbidly obese people found SIBO in seventeen per cent of subjects (compared to 2.5 per cent in non-obese people)[109].

With SIBO being a contributing factor in several common disorders, a test might be wise if you suffer from fatty stools, lactose intolerance, B12 deficient anaemia, alternate constipation and diarrhoea, gas, bloating, and flatulence.

What's involved in taking this test?

This test measures levels of hydrogen and methane in the breath after ingestion of lactulose. You are required to provide twelve breath samples collected over three hours, either at home or in the laboratory where you are taking the test. If there is a peak in the breath before ninety minutes (i.e. if the bacteria of the small intestine are producing excessive by products due to fermentation) this would represent a positive result. No food and or drink except water are allowed for fourteen hours prior to the test.

Helicobacter Pylori Stool Test

Helicobacter pylori is a bacterial infection that is strongly associated with increased risk of stomach or duodenal ulcers. If you suffer from indigestion, gastritis, heartburn, a lot of burping, heart disease, ulcers, reflux, nausea, decreased appetite, bloated stomach, or if there's a family member with gastric cancer, it would be worth considering this test.

What's involved in taking this test?

Stool samples are taken in your own home over the course of three consecutive days and then couriered to the laboratory.

Intestinal Permeability Urine Test

Leaky gut could well be a problem where inflammatory bowel disease (IBD) such as Crohn's or ulcerative colitis are present, or when any of the following ailments are present; food allergy, inflammatory joint disease, skin conditions such as psoriasis and eczema or autoimmune rheumatoid arthritis or ankylosing spondylitis. Not only can this test help with initial diagnosis it can also be used to predict relapses in already established illnesses. A study published in *The Lancet* found that the leaky gut test could be used as an accurate predictor of relapse when measured in patients with Crohn's disease who were clinically in remission[110]

What's involved in taking this test?

Fasting is required for just three hours before starting the test. The test requires a six hour urine collection after a 3g oral dose of a non-toxic substance called

PEG (polyethylene glycol). After swallowing the PEG, a limited amount of water is consumed so as to make sure the urine collected is concentrated enough to trace whether products that should not be present are present thereby indicating leaky gut.

Intestinal Permeability Blood Test

This test looks at the integrity of the gut lining, the presence of bacterial toxins, and tight-junction proteins such as zonulin – high levels of which may indicate the presence of openings between the gut lining and the bloodstream. It identifies both transcellular (through the cells) and paracellular (between the cells) routes of intestinal barrier penetration (leaky gut) by large molecules with a capacity to challenge the immune system. Claude Andre, the leading French research worker in this area, has proposed that measurement of gut permeability is a sensitive and practical screening test for the presence of food allergy. In fact, at the Hospital St. Vincent de Paul in Paris, permeability testing has been effectively used with allergic infants to determine which dietary modifications their mothers needed to

Cellular penetration of antigens

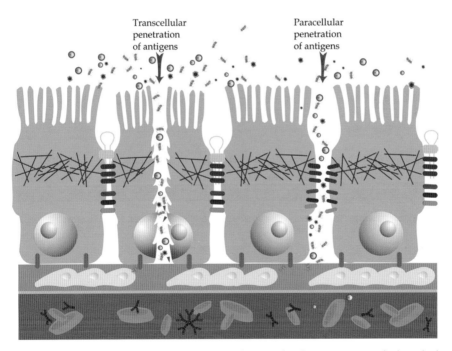

Intestinal permeability tests look at the two routes large molecules can penetrate the intestinal barrier i.e. between the cells or through the cells.

make while breastfeeding and which of the 'hypoallergenic' infant formulas they needed to avoid in order to relieve their symptoms[111].

This test is recommended for those who present with multiple symptom complaints (including unexplained fatigue), suffer from abnormal immune cell count and function (including autoimmune diseases) and those who complain of food allergy and intolerance

What's involved in taking this test?
This is a blood test which needs to be carried out by a doctor or phlebotomist who will take your blood and centrifuge it, before it is sent off to a laboratory.

In summary, there are several tests available to help people understand what their digestive issue is. It would be recommended that you work with a suitably qualified health practitioner to work out which is the most suitable test for your digestive complaint or health history. Many people are digestively asymptomatic and have no digestive-related symptoms but the root of their health issue is in fact a digestive one. Identifying the cause would be a step in the direction of finding a solution.

Chapter 13

Autism and Gut Health

Autism cases have increased almost six-fold over the past twenty years and both scientists and parents have begun to question why. Although many experts point to environmental factors, others have focused on changes to the microbiome. Children with autism are far more likely to have digestive problems than those without the disorder[112]. In one study, eighty-five per cent of children on the autistic spectrum were diagnosed with constipation[113]. According to one report, more than ninety per cent of children with autism spectrum disorders suffer from chronic, severe gastrointestinal symptoms. Gastrointestinal issues appear to be linked to autism-related problems, including issues with social interaction, irritability and repetitive behaviours.

Healthy and abnormal CNS and gut function

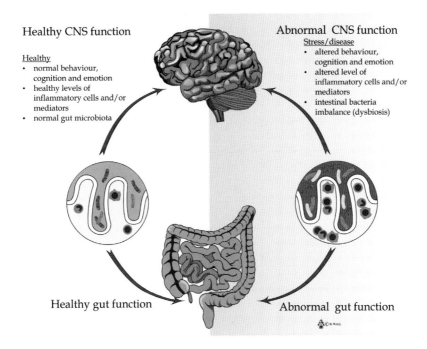

Healthy CNS function

Healthy
- normal behaviour, cognition and emotion
- healthy levels of inflammatory cells and/or mediators
- normal gut microbiota

Abnormal CNS function
Stress/disease
- altered behaviour, cognition and emotion
- altered level of inflammatory cells and/or mediators
- intestinal bacteria imbalance (dysbiosis)

Healthy gut function

Abnormal gut function

Are the gut bacteria of autistic people different?

There is evidence to suggest that the gut bacteria in children with autism do vary from those of children without it. Potentially pathogenic forms of the bacteria clostridium are found in autistic people in greater numbers. Clostridium bolteae was discovered in 2003. It is known to play a role in gastrointestinal disorders, and it often shows up in higher numbers in the gastrointestinal tracts of autistic children than in those of other children[114]. In a 2005 study, scientists looked at the stools of autistic children, and found that the flora of ASD (autistic spectrum disorder) patients contained a higher incidence of the clostridium histolyticum group of bacteria. The problem with having higher levels of these bacteria is that they're not only recognised toxin-producers, but the products of these toxins are thought to have a systemic effect on health.[115] This may explain why autism presents as an ailment affecting behaviours, mood and social skills, and not simply the gut.

The composition of bacteria in the intestines is often abnormal in people with autism. The obvious question is whether digestive problems and microbial differences are the reason for the development of the condition or are instead a consequence of it. We must consider that any pre-existing digestion or bowel-related problems may be exacerbated by autistic behaviour. People with autism can sometimes develop very strong food preferences, such as only eating one type of food, or only food of a certain colour, which can itself produce bowel problems. A study published in December 2013[116] supports the argument that autism develops as a result of microbial differences. Researchers at the California Institute of Technology infected pregnant mice with a mock virus. The immune system spikes after the mock virus injection and autism-like symptoms result in the offspring such as obsessive grooming and a disinterest in other mice. The researchers found that after birth, the infected mice had altered gut bacteria compared to healthy mice. Within the same study, the researchers also realised that the health-promoting bacterium bacteroides fragilis could improve some of the behavioural symptoms of those infected via their mothers. The treated mice had less anxious behaviours and became more vocally communicative. Two important lessons from this study are that maternal infection alters the microbiome in their young and probiotics may help reduce the severity of autism-like symptoms in offspring.

In another study by two scientists from Arizona State's Biodesign Unit, it was discovered that children with autism had a greatly reduced spectrum of gut bacteria. One in particular, Prevotella, was missing completely whilst the researchers found that the children with autism seemed to be missing hundreds of beneficial gut bacteria.[117] In other studies, autistic children have been found to have lower levels of bifidobacterium. One particular study[118] found not only bifidobacterium was low but also another bacterium called Akkermansia muciniphila. Low levels of these bacteria have been linked to low levels of antimicrobial molecules in response to an pathogenic invader in the intestine[119] which could help to explain a link between autism and gut health - that children with gut health issues and autism are unable to fight off pathogenic invaders. Once the pathogenic invaders take hold they can play a role in systemic ill-health.

Probiotics as a treatment for autism

We have already discovered that bacteroides fragilis improved autistic symptoms in a study on mice. Now a spate of new studies suggests that restoring proper microbial balance could alleviate some of autism's behavioural symptoms. Perhaps one of the most pertinent studies was one that was a victim of its own success. The study ran in 2006 at the University of Reading. In this study, forty autistic children between the ages of four and thirteen were

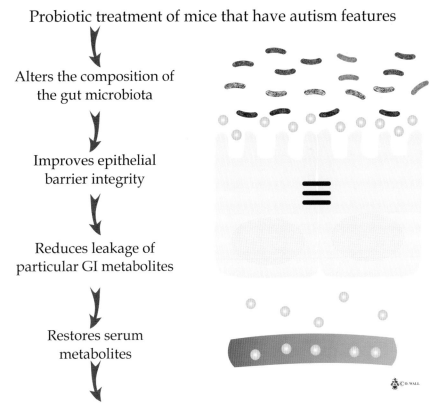

Probiotic treatment of mice that have autism features

↓

Alters the composition of the gut microbiota

↓

Improves epithelial barrier integrity

↓

Reduces leakage of particular GI metabolites

↓

Restores serum metabolites

↓

Ameliorates specific autism-related behavioral abnormalities

In research probiotics have been shown to ameliorate specific autism-related behaviours.

separated into two groups. The first group were given a probiotic supplement, L. plantarum, whilst the other group were given placebos. After three weeks, the two groups were supposed to switch over, the first group would move to the placebos and the second would be given the L. plantarum. However, it seems that the probiotics had such a positive effect on the participants that parents soon realised which group they were in and those whose children were being given the probiotics refused to go into the control group. Parents of children receiving the probiotics could see noticeable differences in their children's health. As a result, participants began to drop out of the study so they could try and replicate the probiotic supplementation themselves. The beneficial effects reported included improved digestive health (including better formed stools) as well as behavioural improvements, with some parents noting that their children were more calm and relaxed and less stressed, and one set of parents even observed that the probiotics had, 'improved ability to listen and concentrate'.[120]

MMR, vaccines and gut health

The link between the MMR vaccine and gut health is one of such notoriety and media speculation thanks mostly to one person who stated that he saw a link between the MMR vaccine and gut problems. That person was Andrew Wakefield. In an article in *The Lancet* in 1998, Andrew Wakefield along with eleven other authors noted that a condition called ILNH (inflammation of the lymph nodes in the gut) co-existed in children with impaired learning skills. This was based on a very small population of just twelve children. It was noted that in eight cases, the parents or the children's doctors made a link between the onset of ILNH and the MMR.[121] This study has subsequently been retracted and Andrew Wakefield has been very much in the media spotlight for many years after being struck off the medical register by the General Medical Council in the UK. The link between gastrointestinal problems and autism is not in itself support for the existence of a link between MMR and autism. The Wakefield study was unable to prove that gastrointestinal upset preceded the MMR vaccine in those affected. In fact what studies show is that gastrointestinal problems exist in autistic children who have never had the MMR vaccine.

However, the correlation between poor gut health markers and vaccine may not be as far-fetched as some believe. That's because the state and composition of the microbiome may ultimately affect how well vaccines work. Studies exploring the relationship between the microbiome and our immune system are raising some interesting findings that may influence the way vaccines are administered to people depending on their gut health and composition in the future. The scientists responsible for two studies looking at the response to vaccines in relation to microbiome diversity discovered that greater diversity in the gut microbiota enables a more robust immune response to vaccines.[122, 123]

A further study entitled 'Influence of the microbiota on vaccine effectiveness' started with researchers giving mice a flu vaccine and antibiotics. Of course the antibiotics killed off the 'good' bacteria so that the researchers could compare the effects of the vaccine on a gut populated with a diverse range of bacteria (a 'good gut') versus a gut without a range of bacteria or with very low levels (a 'bad gut'). What they found was that the mice that had been treated with the microbe-killing antibiotic did not have the same antibody response to the vaccine. In other words, they saw a large drop in how well the vaccine worked. The researchers found the same issue with the polio vaccine. This study was carried out on mice but if the relationship between intestinal bacteria and vaccine effectiveness also held true in humans it has some interesting implications. We know that a young child's immune system and gut diversity is still developing when they are administered under the NHS ten different vaccines before the age of two. The question is whether gut microbiome health should be assessed prior to vaccine. A further question then might be that if poor gut health is linked to poor response to vaccines, then could probiotics help?

Probiotics and vaccines

It seems that the administration of probiotics prior to vaccination could improve how well the vaccine works by boosting the immune system. In one study, both lactobacilli and bifidobacterium were shown to enhance the effectiveness of a vaccine against human rotavirus.[124] Whilst multiple other studies[125] show that using probiotics in the weeks leading up to vaccines to boost the immune system can result in reduced side effects.

In summary, there is most definitely a link between gut health and autism and it appears to be a causal relationship with poor gut health preceding autism. Selective use of probiotics can be used to improve symptoms of autism by addressing poor gut health. Finally, poor gut health and vaccines are also linked. Once again, studies show that supplementing with probiotics in advance of vaccine administration may help the vaccine to work and reduce the likelihood or severity of side effects.

Chapter 14

The Gut-Brain Axis

Although a relatively new area of study[126], as recently as 2009 scientists made a clear connection between gut bacteria and brain activity. The actual anatomical link between the two areas is a long nerve called the vagus nerve. Understanding the critical role that this nerve plays in the processes involved in our overall health and wellbeing is key to understanding just how closely the gut and the brain are linked. We'll be exploring that link in this chapter.

This close relationship between the gut and brain can be seen from our earliest days. When we are babies, a lot of what we feel is down to the gut or the brain and the connection between the two. We love that feeling of being satisfied by a belly full of milk, but we don't like tummy pains, trapped wind or getting cold or wet, and sure enough one part of the body soon lets the other know it

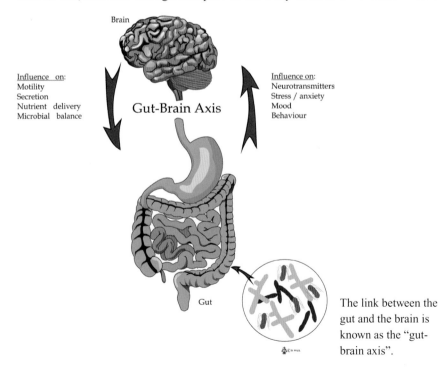

Brain

Influence on:
Motility
Secretion
Nutrient delivery
Microbial balance

Gut-Brain Axis

Influence on:
Neurotransmitters
Stress / anxiety
Mood
Behaviour

Gut

The link between the gut and the brain is known as the "gut-brain axis".

isn't happy with a scream or a cry. As we grow up, the connection between the gut and the brain becomes marginally more refined but we know from multiple studies that a well-nourished gut provides us with optimal wellbeing.

The evidence is building that not only is poor brain health linked to the microbiome but that rectifying the microbiome might benefit brain health and functioning. One 2015 study[127] provided patients without mood disorders with a multi-strain probiotic. After four weeks, those taking the probiotic showed a significantly reduced overall reaction to sadness, which meant less deep thought and fewer aggressive instincts. Another study, carried out in 2013[128], showed that people who consumed a fermented yogurt containing specific probiotics, twice a day for four weeks, experienced changes to their brain when tested at the end of the study. The responses to an emotion recognition task were far better for those who had consumed the yogurt versus those who had not. It seems that the positive outcome is related to the bacteria strains in the yogurt and their effects on the gut, which in turn positively influences the signals sent from the gut to the brain.

When we refer to what has now become known as the 'gut-brain axis' we are in fact talking about the communication between the hormone (endocrine) system and the messenger (nervous) system. There are about 500 million neurons in your gut. These neurons help control your digestion and they also communicate with your brain via the vagus nerve to ensure your physical and mental wellbeing.

Can probiotics help your brain function and improve your mood?

Both human and animal studies show a very close connection between the gut and the brain and the positive outcome of probiotic supplementation on the functioning of them both. One such example is the forced swimming test carried out on mice. In this experiment, a mouse is placed in a small container of water that is too deep for it to reach the bottom. The question is how long does the mouse swim around in the hope of finding a way out before giving up? The answer depends on how prone to depression that mouse is. In older tests, mice fed antidepressants swam for longer. However in one, more recent, study[129] half of the mice were fed the probiotic L. rhamnosus JB-1. The mice in the forced swimming test fed with the probiotic swam for longer than the mice without and scientists also measured less stress hormones in the blood of the probiotic supplemented mice. Mice also performed better in memory and learning tests when fed this probiotic. However, when the vagus nerve in both mice with probiotics and those without was cut, the outcome for both groups was the same. This indicates that the communicating mechanism or route between the gut and the brain is the vagus nerve.

In order to understand the vagus nerve link between the gut and the brain it is important to understand that the vast majority of the output of our brain (about ninety per cent) goes into the lower part of the brain stem which goes into the vagus nerve. Vagus is Latin for 'wandering 'and this is a true description of this nerve, which emerges at the back of the skull and meanders its way through the abdomen, with a number of branching nerves coming into contact with other body parts including the gut. One of the first signs of a poorly functioning brain is low vagus nerve activity. Where digestion is concerned, this can manifest itself as a decrease in digestive enzymes, and lower amounts of bile, which we know can help break down fats, as the activity of the gallbladder, which releases the bile, slows down. As the vagus nerve is linked to the gut, lower vagus nerve activity can affect the immune system and blood flow in the gut. This is an opportunity for pathogenic yeast and bacteria to grow unchallenged. Both yeast and bacteria overgrowth can contribute to intestinal permeability (or leaky gut) which in turn can cause a state of inflammation. Inflammatory messengers called cytokines are then produced in the gut and travel through the brain transported in the blood across the blood-brain barrier. One of the problems with inflammation is that it makes the blood-brain barrier more permeable so you get 'leaky brain' happening too. Then those inflammatory cytokines, once they get into the brain, activate the immune cells, leading to inflammation of the brain. This is linked to depression as the rate at which messages are sent declines, resulting in a reduction of vagus nerve activity. You can see how this cycle becomes self-perpetuating.

Can we take probiotics for depression?

The evidence is stacking up that gut health is certainly linked to mental health and that in many studies the supplementation of probiotics has improved depressive or low mood symptoms. A study carried out in 2007[130] found that drinking a probiotic milk drink for three weeks improved the mood of those who initially had the lowest mood. In 2009, a study[131] carried out on people with chronic fatigue syndrome found that supplementing with L. casei significantly reduced self-reported anxiety. In this particular example, the supplementation of L. casei seemed to boost the host's levels of both lactobacillus and bifidobacterium. This supports evidence that supplementing some strains of probiotics can provide a favourable environment for others to thrive. More and more studies have proved this positive association between probiotic supplementation and better mental health and wellbeing. Furthermore, a study carried out on petrochemical workers in 2015[132] linked the consumption of either a probiotic yogurt or a probiotic capsule with improved mental wellbeing too.

Finally, and I think this sums up where we are today in relation to gut health and probiotics boosting mental health and wellbeing, this 2016[133] study concluded that, 'Although an association between gut health and certain psychiatric conditions has long been recognised, it now appears that gut microbes represent direct mediators of psychopathology.' This statement implies that there is a pressing need for microbiome testing in diagnosing disorders associated with the brain.

In summary, gut health and brain health have been shown to be linked. Low mood is directly related to poor microbiome status. Testing could be deployed as part of the suite of diagnostic tools used in brain disorders. Probiotics have been shown to improve mood and depressive symptoms and this advance in our knowledge should be what informs the treatment of mood disorders in the future. Added to this, we need more diagnostic screening of the gut when we are looking to treat brain disorders.

Chapter 15

Eczema and Gut Health

What is eczema?

Eczema is a broad selection of skin conditions characterised by dry skin, rashes and itching. Although there are many types of eczema, the one with a direct link to gut flora and diet is known as atopic eczema. Atopic eczema is a chronic skin condition and an allergic disease that tends to be passed down from generation to generation. It is known to occur along with other allergic diseases such as asthma, hay fever and food allergy. There is evidence to link eczema with gastrointestinal diseases involving food intolerance.

How does gut health affect skin health?

Gut bacterial balance affects many different areas of health, but one of the most important to consider is how the establishment of bacterial balance during early childhood is linked to the development of atopic diseases such as eczema, asthma and allergies. Although atopic conditions are often passed down from generation to generation there's also a steady rise in the number of children suffering. In fact eczema now affects one in ten American infants and children[134] and between fifteen and thirty per cent of children in the UK.[135] Healthy gut balance during early life protects against these conditions. Gut balance during infancy is dependent on a number of factors, including: the birthing method (C-Section or via the birthing canal), diet of the mother both whilst pregnant and during breastfeeding and the administration of probiotics or antibiotics to both the child and mother. This early gut microbial development primes immune function and that priming can have lifelong protective and preventative effects on health.

Research suggests that the microbial balance of those diagnosed with atopic diseases may not be 'optimal'. What we expect of a good balance is to include a large amount of beneficial bacteria, such as bifidobacterium and lactobacillus species, and a minimal amount of potential pathogens. What's been discovered in the guts of those who have atopic diseases is of great interest. Whilst it is largely agreed that infants prone to eczema have less probiotic bacteria naturally present they also have less diversity. Clostridium difficile, a pathogenic bacterium, has been found in the guts of babies with an increased probability of eczema, asthma and allergic sensitivity.[136] It has also been discovered that children who suffer from atopic diseases are more likely to be depleted of certain immune-boosting species too. The reasons for this can only be hypothesised at this stage but the hypotheses include:

1. Dietary factors – including length of breastfeeding
2. Birth method
3. Use of antibiotics in infancy

It seems that children breastfed for longer are less likely to suffer from atopic diseases. Those born via the birthing canal are also less vulnerable and children who have not been administered with antibiotics early on have a better chance of escaping atopic illness too. We know that all three of these factors may contribute to optimal bacterial balance in the gut.

Eczema-Gluten Link

Eczema is also commonly diagnosed in people with coeliac disease and those with non-coeliac gluten sensitivity. Researchers have compared the prevalence of eczema in people who also suffer from coeliac disease to eczema prevalence in control subjects, and they've found that eczema occurs about three times more frequently in coeliac disease patients and about two times more frequently in the relatives of coeliac disease patients, indicating that there may be a genetic link between the two conditions[137].

Although non-coeliac gluten sensitivity is still not as well understood as coeliac disease, it has also been associated with eczema. Symptoms of non-coeliac gluten sensitivity include digestive issues (such as diarrhoea, constipation, pain and bloating), plus other symptoms, including brain fog and skin conditions connected to gluten consumption. One 2015 study[138] looked at 17 people with non-coeliac gluten sensitivity who had skin problems, including rashes that looked like eczema, dermatitis herpetiformis and psoriasis. The study found that the skin of these people improved significantly within one month of adopting a gluten free diet.

Do probiotics heal eczema?

One of the earliest studies to show how effective specific probiotic strains could be in lowering the risk of atopic disease was published in 2000[139]. For this study, the researchers studied 27 babies who had been diagnosed with atopic eczema despite the fact they were exclusively breastfed. The babies were divided into three groups.

Group 1: Placebo
Group 2: Receiving the probiotic lactobacillus GG
Group 3: Receiving the probiotic bifidobacterium lactis.

The result was that groups two and three (which received the probiotic supplements), improved significantly while the placebo group did not. This isn't a lone study. More evidence of the positive effects of probiotics in treating atopic dermatitis was provided by a 2003 study. In this study[140], the combination of two strains of lactobacillus (L. rhamnosus and L. reuteri) was given to children aged between one and thirteen years for six weeks. The researchers used the SCORAD (scoring atopic dermatitis) index to determine the effectiveness of the probiotics. The results of this study showed that fifty-six per cent of the children who were given the two probiotic strains got better, but only fifteen per cent of the placebo group improved. In this study, the researchers also found that probiotics were more effective for eczema patients who also had positive skin prick test response (a test of allergen sensitivity). People with allergy sensitive eczema (also known as IgE-associated eczema) typically test positive for an airborne or food-based sensitivity and the probiotic supplementation seemed to help improve their eczema symptoms.

A later study carried out in 2007[141] specifically investigated whether probiotics can help prevent IgE-associated eczema. The study involved 188 pregnant women. These women were selected as they came from families with a history of allergic diseases and a very high risk of IgE-associated eczema. Some of the women were given the probiotic supplement L. reuteri from week 36 of their pregnancy until delivery. Thereafter, the babies born from those women were given the same probiotic from birth until they were twelve months old. The results of the study showed that the babies from the probiotic group had significantly lower rates of IgE-associated eczema. What's more is that the protection offered by the probiotic treatment was still effective twelve months later and even though they were no longer taking the probiotics.

Are all probiotics as good as each other in treating eczema?

Although the evidence suggests that probiotic supplementation or at least increasing the levels of 'good' bacteria in the gut of pregnant women and breastfed babies (via mother's milk) is a positive step in the prevention or reduction in eczema, it is also clear that not all probiotics and in fact prebiotics are equal when it comes to atopic disease. In one study, researchers compared the effectiveness of two different probiotic strains to a placebo in the prevention of atopic eczema. They divided pregnant women into three groups. Whilst one group was given a placebo, the other two groups were given either L. rhamnosus or B. animalis. The pregnant women followed these treatments from five weeks before their due dates to six months after their babies were delivered, as long as they were still breastfeeding. Their babies also received three treatments before the age of two. The results showed that L. rhamnosus significantly reduced the incidence of eczema compared to the placebo. However, this was not the case with the B. animalis strain.

How can prebiotics be used in the treatment of eczema?

Prebiotics are fibres that cannot be absorbed or broken down by the body and therefore serve as a great food source for probiotics. In theory, if probiotics are able to help prevent or reduce the incidence of eczema then prebiotics, the food source of probiotics, should also be able to boost the effectiveness of the probiotics in improving the outcome of intervention. Certainly, there are studies that concur with this.

One 2007 study[142] compared a mixture of prebiotics and four probiotic strains to a placebo in the prevention of atopic eczema. The researchers gave over 1,200 pregnant women either a placebo or the mixture of probiotics and prebiotics during their last months of pregnancy. Then they gave the same treatment to their babies for six months. After two years, the results showed that the mixture of probiotics and prebiotics reduced the incidence of IgE-related eczema and also increased the population of lactobacillus and bifidobacteria species in the gut of the infants. This suggests that a combination of probiotics and prebiotics could help reduce the incidence of eczema if women start to use this combination whilst still pregnant and if their babies then used it in the first six months of life.

How are gut health and eczema linked?

What appears to be clear is that gut bacterial balance plays a huge part in the likelihood of eczema. Multiple factors, including the diet of the mother before birth and whilst breastfeeding; the length of breastfeeding; the birth method and the administration of antibiotics can all play a part in how likely it is that people will suffer from eczema. Certainly many studies have also shown that the supplementation with probiotics during pregnancy and supplementing the baby up to twelve months of age may help to decrease the chances of suffering from eczema. Furthermore, a combination of prebiotics and probiotics may help in the fight against eczema as could following a gluten free diet if there are other markers of gluten sensitivity.

Chapter 16

Food Allergy and Gut Health

We know that in just one generation, a change in the prevalence of food allergy and food anaphylaxis has occurred. It seems most likely that something has been changing in our environment to bring this about, and that this has directly or indirectly affected gut health, which is of course an integral part of the immune system. We know that the overuse of antibiotics and diets rich in processed foods have changed the composition of the bacteria in our intestines but why would those changes not apply to everyone? Why are there some people who are allergic to a given food while other people are not? The answer could be related to differences in the gut bacteria of allergic individuals.

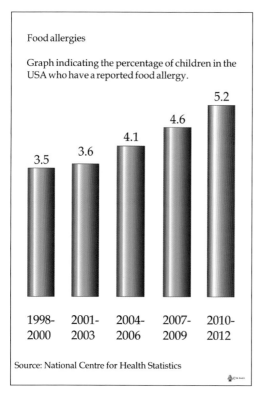

Food allergies

Graph indicating the percentage of children in the USA who have a reported food allergy.

3.5 — 1998-2000
3.6 — 2001-2003
4.1 — 2004-2006
4.6 — 2007-2009
5.2 — 2010-2012

Source: National Centre for Health Statistics

The number of children with food allergy is rising year on year.

Gut bacteria and food allergy

Alterations in gut bacteria have been found in infants suffering from allergy. In general, allergic children appear to have a delayed development of lactobacillus and bifidobacterium. Some scientists now suggest that a lack of exposure to the microbes in the environment as babies is linked to a rising frequency of allergy. Some supporting evidence for this is derived from the fact that C-section babies are at increased risk of food allergy. This suggests that early colonisation of the digestive tract with the right kind of microbes might build tolerance to food allergens.

Can probiotics or prebiotics be used to treat food allergy?

Probiotics and prebiotics are regularly being studied as a means of both prevention and treatment of atopic diseases (eczema, asthma and allergy). However, most of the clinical trials using probiotics have examined their effects on eczema and only a few studies have examined their effect on food allergy. Whilst more studies have been carried out on mice than humans, the findings so far are promising. In one study,[143] rebalancing gut microbes led to greater tolerance to allergens, but importantly, this was only the case in infants and not adults. However, from all of the research available it appears that the supplementation of probiotics for the treatment of food allergy is far more complex than simply buying an over the counter probiotic and hoping for an allergy free life.

From the animal-based studies it has been found that a probiotic mixture of eight different bacterial strains (L. acidophilus, L. delbrueckii, L. casei, L. plantarum, B. longum. B. infantis, B. breve, and Streptococcus salivarius) could decrease the severity of the reaction to the allergenic food and reduce the amount of histamine in the stools. This effect was associated with a decrease in levels of inflammatory cytokines and an increase in the levels of regulatory cytokines. Cytokines, of course, being chemical messengers that tell the body how to react to a particular substance.[144]

In another study[145] the researchers exposed germ-free mice (born and raised in sterile conditions so that they had no native gut bacteria) and mice treated with antibiotics as newborns (which we know significantly reduces gut bacteria) to peanut allergens. Both groups of mice displayed a strong immune system response, producing significantly higher levels of antibodies to fight the peanut allergens than mice with a normal population of gut bacteria. However, the researchers found that this sensitisation to food allergens could be reversed by reintroducing a mix of Clostridia bacteria into the mice's guts. The researchers did further tests which revealed that the Clostridia appeared to make the gut less leaky in allergic mice. Work is underway to create probiotic supplements containing Clostridia.

One trial of lactobacillus GG infant formula compared to formula alone demonstrated that those on the supplemented formula developed tolerance to cow's milk at a faster rate.[146]

Straight supplementation of probiotics is one thing but now probiotics are also being used as a delivery mechanism for other benefits. In the case of food allergies, probiotics are being used to send food antigens (these have been engineered to ensure an immune response from the body once they reach their destination) into the body, to reach areas that can only be reached by using probiotics as the delivery mechanism. Once there, the antigen can cause the body to respond favourably to an allergenic food when the body is next exposed to that food. In this way probiotics may be helpful in reducing the number of people suffering from life-threatening food allergies. Results from rodent studies have been extremely positive. They show an increased tolerance to milk and eggs where probiotics have been engineered to express milk and egg antigens. Each of the animal-based studies provides evidence to suggest that this method could either treat or prevent sensitization to the food antigen being administered by bringing about a change in the immune response. This area of study is in its infancy but it is extremely promising given the rise in numbers of food allergy sufferers in recent years and our increasing knowledge of probiotics.

Instead of engineering lacotcoccus lactis to express an antigen, some researchers have engineered the bacteria to induce regulatory cytokines in order to tolerate allergenic food and drink.[147, 148, 149] This method has also been shown to reduce anaphylaxis scores. There is some further evidence to suggest that treatment with two different strains of lacotcoccus lactis, one expressing a cytokine and the other expressing the food antigen of interest, could lead to a synergistic effect not obtained by administering either alone. Although these methods provide insight into what may be possible in the future they have yet to be studied extensively in humans. Only when this is done, will we know if they could be used on allergic individuals to reduce the severity of their anaphylaxis.

In summary, whilst there are alterations in the gut bacteria of allergic children there is no direct link between probiotic supplementation and reduction in food allergy. However, probiotics may be used as a delivery mechanism to trick the immune system into reducing the reaction to a food allergen. This is a promising development and an area to watch for developments.

Chapter 17

Stress, Sleep and Gut Bugs

I just want real reactions. I want people to laugh from the gut, be sad from the gut - or get angry from the gut - Andy Kaufman

Our gut communicates with multiple cells in the body, which means that disturbances in the gut can show up as disturbances in the brain (and vice versa). As a matter of fact, the brain actually kicks off digestion before the gut because we secrete acids and digestive enzymes before even swallowing the first bite of a meal.

The Gut is the 'Seat of Emotions'

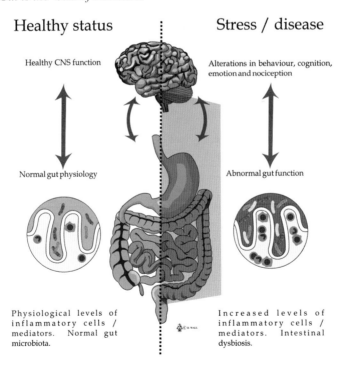

Healthy status / Stress / disease

Healthy CNS function

Alterations in behaviour, cognition, emotion and nociception

Normal gut physiology

Abnormal gut function

Physiological levels of inflammatory cells / mediators. Normal gut microbiota.

Increased levels of inflammatory cells / mediators. Intestinal dysbiosis.

The effects of stress and disease on the bacterial balance and functioning of the gut.

Our emotions can also influence the health of our gut. When you're afraid, your brain and gut registers this, and your digestion slows down. Have you ever had the experience of not being able to eat when you're feeling especially anxious? A lot of people will feel this sensation just before a big competition or exam.

trust your gut - anon

When we are resting and not stressed the gut receives a good flow of blood, but during periods of stress, blood flow to the gut can drop significantly. Lack of blood flow to the gut during digestion can slow down the process, resulting in food hanging around in the gut and an increased risk of intestinal permeability (leaky gut).

The effect of stress on your digestion.

The gut is especially vulnerable to the presence of stress. When we are under stress, our body produces less stomach acid (also known as 'hydrochloric acid'), our digestive system works more slowly than normal and the subsequent effect is often intestinal permeability induced food intolerance. Food intolerance levels have risen significantly in recent years and many would argue that this coincides with our lives becoming more and more stressful, thanks to our "always on", 24/7 culture and work habits.

Stomach acid and stress

Having too little stomach acid is a condition known as 'hypochlorydia'. Stomach acid declines with stress, age and the use of certain medications. Low stomach acid level manifests itself in many ways including:

- Indigestion, especially after a protein-rich meal
- Food intolerances
- Bloating
- Belching
- Burning
- Flatulence immediately after meals
- Feeling full after meals for longer than normal
- Diarrhoea or constipation
- Undigested foods in stools
- Anaemia
- Poor hair or nail health

Why is low stomach acid a problem?

1. We need proper levels of stomach acid to absorb nutrients including minerals (iron, copper, zinc and calcium), vitamin B12, folic acid and proteins.
2. Stomach acid also forms an important part of the immune system and helps form a barrier that kills bacteria and other bugs that enter the body.

Why reflux or acid stomach might be low stomach acid not too much acid?

Insufficient stomach acid can lead to an increase in intra-abdominal pressure (IAP). When IAP increases, the stomach pushes against the lower sphincter in the oesophagus. When the sphincter opens due to the pressure and acid touches the inside of the oesophagus, it hurts. There's a sensation of pain and burning. This is because the oesophagus is not protected like the stomach from high acid levels. The oesophagus was never designed to come into contact with acid.

Gastric reflux

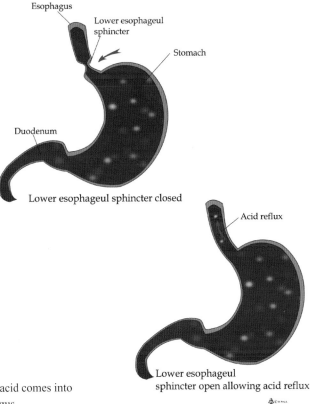

When acid reflux occurs acid comes into contact with the oesophagus.

If you experience wind or bloating after a meal it is likely that food is being fermented by bacteria. If your acid levels are low enough and bacteria are surviving in the stomach repeated burps after eating are likely. Sometimes, tasting your meal again several hours after eating can be a sign that the food is still in your stomach when it should be in your small intestine.

How to find out if you have low stomach acid?

You can use bicarbonate of soda, an alkaline substance, to get an idea of the levels of acid production in your stomach. You simply measure the reaction of the bicarbonate of soda with your stomach acid by the rate at which you burp after consuming the drink.

- Mix together a solution of ¼ tsp bicarbonate of soda and 230ml of cold water.
- After drinking the solution (first thing in the morning and on an empty stomach), measure the amount of time it takes before you burp:
  - 2-3 mins = adequate stomach acid
  - Less than 2 mins or if you continue to burp = too much stomach acid
  - 5 minutes = too little stomach acid

What to do if you have low stomach acid?

The first thing you can do if your stomach acid levels are low is to ensure that you do not drink water at mealtimes. Try and drink water up to thirty minutes before and an hour after meals and throughout the day in between meals. This ensures that you are not diluting the stomach acid you produce while eating but you still maintain a level of hydration sufficient to encourage good digestion. Secondly, you should try to reduce or limit the amount of stress in your life whenever and wherever this is possible. Thirdly, if your stomach acid levels are extremely low you can use apple cider vinegar to help your body recognise the need to produce more of its own stomach acid in order to break down food efficiently. Follow this process for introducing apple cider vinegar:

- Add 1 teaspoon of apple cider vinegar to water and drink with each meal.
- Gradually increase with each meal.
- If you experience burning neutralise with 1 tsp bicarbonate of soda in water or milk.
- Take 1 less teaspoonful until burning stops.

Over time, your stomach will begin to produce its own stomach acid again so you will not be taking the same dose forever. As soon as you feel a burning sensation, reduce the dosage until eventually your stomach is producing all of the acid it needs.

How does stress affect our overall health via the gut?

There is evidence to suggest that gut bacteria may respond negatively to stress, leaving our body more prone to infection, pathogens and digestive problems. If you have ever heard of people suffering from a 'nervous stomach' or a 'gut feeling' then you will probably not be surprised to find out that there is a very close relationship between these sensations and activity in the brain. The gut is an integral part of the nervous system. The biochemical changes that occur in times of stress have significant and immediate effects on your gut function. The process of stress can cause inflammation, increase gut permeability (leaky gut), heighten your perception of pain and raise gut motility (how quickly food is processed and moved through your system.) Furthermore, chronic exposure to stress may lead to the development of a variety of gastrointestinal diseases including:

1. Gastroesophageal reflux disease (GERD)
2. Peptic ulcers
3. IBD - ulcerative colitis and Crohn's disease
4. IBS
5. Food allergy

Whilst poor dietary choices can lead to further stress on our system so can unwise lifestyle choices. Overtraining, insufficient sleep or even not including enough 'you time' or pleasure-giving activities in your own life can make stress levels far worse. Stress can cause your body to produce stress hormones at too high a level which is unsustainable and may ultimately end with fatigue. Stress hormone patterns can lead to weight gain, sleep disturbances, and even a reduction in life span.

Sleep and gut bugs

Getting enough sleep is important to allow your body time for rest and repair. As well as this, prolonged periods of insufficient sleep have associations with increased risk of disease. Particularly relevant to sleep is something called our circadian rhythm. That's the rhythmic way in which our bodies respond to a 24-hour cycle of light and darkness in our environment. Evidence shows that poor sleep cycles actually alter our microbiome and therefore our gut health. Gut bugs have a rhythm too. Each rhythm needs to be in sync with the other. Microbiome rhythms are significantly influenced by dietary choices whilst your circadian rhythm is influenced by a number of factors including lifestyle choices, diet and stress. Insufficient sleep and disruption to the circadian rhythm disrupts the rhythm and balance of the microbiome as well. Furthermore, the microbiome is partially responsible for the production of sleep-regulating neurotransmitters dopamine, serotonin and GABA. A deficiency of the "darkness hormone" melatonin is linked to increased likelihood of leaky gut syndrome, as is an overproduction of stress hormone cortisol.

Could there be a link between poor sleep, obesity and disease risk?

A prolonged lack of sleep also increases cravings for junk food such as refined carbohydrates (white bread, pasta, rice, pies, pasties and cake) as well as sugary foods and drinks. So sleep deprivation may cause an increased consumption of these foods. As refined carbohydrates are known to feed harmful bacteria, this could indirectly lead to poorer gut health. The cycle becomes self-fulfilling. The more junk food is consumed, the poorer energy and sleep levels become, the greater the likelihood of obesity and the greater the chances of an altered microbiome.

Exercise and gut bugs

Over the past few years, a variety of published studies show how exercise exerts a significant positive effect on the health of the microbiome. Looking at the research, it seems that physical activity should be encouraged from an early age if we want optimal gut health for our children. A recent study[150] showed that daily exercise in the young can stimulate the formation of a more beneficial microbial system.

Particularly interesting is one study[151] that presented data on how environmental contaminants can damage the gut microbiome. These detrimental effects are reversed by participation in exercise. The evidence for exercise positively affecting gut health is further supported by this study[152] in which it was shown that athletes show significantly greater microbiome diversity than non-athletes.

In summary, stress, sleep, diet, exercise and the microbiome are all intrinsically linked. Each of these five elements can have a negative onward effect on the other four. We are beginning to understand this interconnectivity more and more and the result is that people are starting to adopt a multi-factorial approach to health. No longer is one area of change enough to achieve optimal health.

Chapter 18

Environmental Chemicals and Gut Health

Whilst the number of health issues stemming from an imbalance of the microbiome is growing so is our understanding of reasons why this may be happening. One causative factor has to be changes to the environment in which we live. That makes sense when populations around the world, their environments and their gut health are analysed. Less polluted and more traditional cultures tend to have much steadier microbiomes, a greater diversity of good bacteria in their guts and less gut-related ill health. In this chapter we'll look at the chemicals that may contribute to gut health problems.

Glyphosate

Around the world, the active ingredient glyphosate is better known as its trade name, the weed killer, Roundup, which you may have seen advertised on television over the years. Glyphosate is not just sold as Roundup however, as it is also used in other weed killers in our parks and green spaces and on playing fields too. Commercially, it is used on a lot of crops grown in fields across Europe and America. Studies have shown that it causes disruption to the way in which our gut microbe's function and how long they survive. Glyphosate may even affect the lifespan of our gut bacteria. In fact, glyphosate seems to have an affinity for attacking beneficial bacteria and allowing pathogens to grow in the gut unopposed. In this way, the presence of glyphosate in the human body has been linked to the rise in the number of cases of the toxic, pathogenic bacteria clostridium botulinum[153]. It has also been linked to a lowering of beneficial bacteria in animals exposed to glyphosate[154].

What's the mechanism for this?

Many claim that glyphosate is harmless to animals and human beings because the mechanism, known as the 'shikimate pathway', that it uses to kill weeds is absent in animals and humans. The problem with that assertion is that bacteria actually have their own shikimate pathway and we have millions of bacteria in our guts. These bacteria are essential to our health. So via the bacteria in our guts it is also possible that exposure to glyphosate could be implicated in immune and digestive problems in humans.

Where is glyphosate used today?

Glyphosate was introduced in the 1970s under the brand Roundup and is the most widely produced weed killer in the world[155]. Although some nations, namely Holland, France and Brazil have already banned the sale of glyphosate over the counter, its global usage continues to grow. In the UK, figures analysed by the Soil Association from government data in 2016 revealed glyphosate use in British farming has increased by 400 per cent in the past twenty years. In the last year for which government figures are available, nearly a third of cereals, wheat and barley in the UK, were sprayed with glyphosate.[156] It will come as no surprise therefore that glyphosate is also the most commonly detected pesticide in loaves of bread. In a review of data gathered by the government in 2013, the Pesticide Action Network (PAN) revealed that traces of at least one pesticide were found in sixty-three per cent of shop-brought loaves, and that contamination has run at these levels for at least a decade. The chemicals were found in bread significantly more frequently than in other foods.

What can we learn from this?

- If you eat grains then choose organic wheat or non-wheat grains.
- Don't use Roundup on your own garden.
- Lobby your local government to stop using glyphosate in public parks and green areas. One local authority that has banned the use of glyphosate is Hammersmith and Fulham[157]. This was only achieved after residents put pressure on the local council.

Artificial sweeteners

Artificial sweeteners are one of the most widely used food additives in the world. Whilst many companies and even governments recommend products containing artificial sweeteners due to their low calorie content, the supporting scientific data remains limited and some studies are emerging that question whether these artificial food additives should be used at all. In one particular study,[158] scientists demonstrated that the consumption of commonly used artificial sweeteners actually affects the bacteria in the gut so that the body becomes even more susceptible to the effects of glucose. That's not good news in the global battle against obesity and diabetes. The problem is that even though artificial sweeteners contain few or no calories they still have to make their way through the gut and it seems that this is where they do the damage. It's here that they seem to favour the growth of bacteria that make more calories available to us and thereby contribute to weight gain.

What can we learn from this?

- Avoid artificial sweeteners.
- Where sweetness is required, try another natural product called pure stevia powder instead. This has a glycaemic index of zero which means it doesn't affect our blood sugar levels.

Antibiotics

There's a whole chapter (Chapter 10) dedicated to the subject of antibiotics and gut health. Many studies suggest that antibiotics can affect gut flora, even changing the microbial and metabolic patterns of the gut.[159] Antibiotics are introduced to our bodies both directly, when we have to take them to eliminate a bacterial infection, and also indirectly, via the consumption of animal produce (the animals involved are dosed up on antibiotics). Livestock, poultry and even fish have routinely been given antibiotics since the 1940s and reports even suggest that more antibiotics are made for animals than humans. The spread of antibiotics becomes even more of an issue when huge quantities of manure are routinely sprayed onto farmers' fields, creating antibiotic resistant bacteria that leech into surface and ground water, contaminating drinking water.

What can we learn from this?

- Only take antibiotics when absolutely necessary.
- When you do have to take antibiotics, also take probiotics although at least two hours away from the antibiotics.
- Try to consume organic and free-range animal products.
- Filter your tap water.

Emulsifiers

Emulsifiers keep the ingredients in processed food from separating and they improve shelf life. However, research[160] shows gut microbiota may be a key direct target of these commonly used food additives. When emulsifiers get into the gut they can ultimately lead to changes in metabolism and also to inflammation. Studies[161] reveal that emulsifiers may cause increased food consumption, obesity and blood sugar imbalance.

What can we learn from this?

- Eat real food. If you are purchasing processed foods then emulsifiers you should look out for on ingredients labels are:
  - ○ Carboxymethyl cellulose (CMC or E466) – used in ice creams, breads, biscuits, chewing gums, margarines and peanut butter.
  - ○ Polysorbate-80 (E433) – used in ice cream, biscuits and chewing gum.

Sugary foods

Not only will overconsumption of sugary foods compromise your beneficial gut bacteria by providing the preferred fuel for invading pathogenic bacteria, it will also contribute to chronic inflammation throughout your body, including your brain. Most processed foods are typically high in refined grains, which turn into sugar in your body. That means they can also provide instant fuel for invading bacteria.

What we can learn from this?

- Try to eliminate processed foods and refined sugars from your diet.

In summary, our gut bacteria can be influenced by both food choices and the environment in which we live. There are steps we can take to minimise our exposure to these microbiome disrupting agents and these steps include reducing exposure to pesticides, artificial sweeteners, antibiotics, emulsifiers and sugary foods.

Chapter 19

Are Gut Microbes to Blame for my Weight?

While we have covered a lot of the connections between gut health and general health, we have not, as yet, discussed how gut health is also related to weight. A recent meta-analysis[162] (where researchers look at the work of a significant number of other scientists on the same subject) found that studies revealed that adding probiotics to your diet can help you lose weight. The study also showed that the more probiotics you take the more weight you'll lose; and that those who take several probiotics a day for at least eight weeks reap the greatest benefits. We are not talking about people shedding stones here, but weight loss could make the difference between someone becoming diabetic or not becoming diabetic so probiotic supplementation is an important consideration here.

The bacteria living in our guts eat what we eat. It is thought that certain microbes (bacteria and fungi) 'crave' particular kinds of food and can communicate this with the brain. This leads to someone making food choices that are influenced by the cravings of the microbes. The most common kind of craving for those with bacteria that are out of balance is for refined carbohydrates such as white bread, cakes, biscuits and sweets. These break down very quickly and easily into a source of energy for those unwelcome microbes in the gut.

Increasing the number of probiotics through supplementation or fermented foods may well broaden the range of foods people with gut problems are willing to try. A better balance of bacteria may lessen unwanted food cravings. Appetites for healthier foods may also return.

Does our microbiome predispose us to obesity?

In one study[163] scientists raised genetically identical baby rodents in a germ free environment so that their bodies would be free of bacteria. Then they introduced to the guts of the rodents the microbes from obese women and their slim twin sisters. The mice ate the same food and in the same quantities and yet the animals that received bacteria from an obese twin grew heavier and had more body fat than mice with microbes from a slim twin. The scientists looked at the diversity of microbes in the guts of the fat mice and found far fewer species of bacteria present. This is exactly what we'd expect to find of course.

However, when the scientists moved the rodents into a shared cage, intriguingly, both groups remained lean. The explanation is that the mice carrying the bacteria from the obese humans actually picked up better, leaner bacteria, varieties of bacteroidetes from the leaner mice by consuming their faeces. It may sound disgusting but that's normal mouse behaviour. What we can learn from this though is that it is possible to change, in fact improve our levels of lean bacteria with an infusion of good bacteria. You'll be pleased to learn that the solution doesn't involve eating poop either.

A.

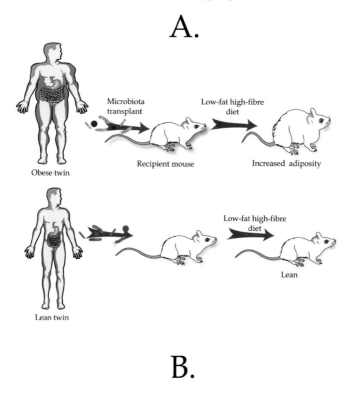

B.

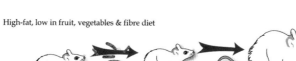

Both diet and environment effect how bacteria play a part in weight gain.

Researchers wanted to prove that an infusion of bacteria can improve weight control so they transferred fifty-four varieties of bacteria from some lean mice to those with the obese type germs and found that the animals that had been destined to become obese developed a healthy weight instead. It has to be said that fifty-four varieties is an awful lot and when the researchers tried the same experiment but transferred just thirty-nine strains, it didn't work. So it seems that research on the ultimate variety of probiotics for weight loss is still needed if our ultimate goal is to be achieved.

These experiments show that diet is an important factor in shaping the gut ecosystem. A diet of highly processed foods, for example, has been linked to a less diverse gut community in people. When the mice in this experiment were fed specially prepared unhealthy food that was high in fat and low in fruits, vegetables and fibre the mice with obese type microbes grew fat even when in the same cage as their lean mates. The unhealthy diet somehow prevented the good bacteria from moving in and thriving.

Antibiotics and body weight

Unfortunately we are now realising that the use of antibiotics may also be linked, via changes to the microbiome, to obesity too. One scientist, Martin Blaser, has shown that when young mice are given low doses of antibiotics, similar to the dose farmers give livestock, they develop about fifteen percent more body fat than mice that are not given these drugs[164]. It is possible that the mechanism for this is that the antibiotics destroy some of the good or lean bacteria that help maintain a healthy weight. Martin Blaser even went on to show a geographical overlap between areas of high antibiotic use and high levels of obesity in humans. He created two maps, one for obesity and one for antibiotic prescriptions per 1000 people. This data from 2010 is enlightening. There is a clear correlation between areas of high antibiotic prescription and areas of high obesity. The opposite is also evident. Where fewer antibiotics are prescribed the obesity levels are also lower.

In summary, weight is affected by gut bacteria. Certain types of gut bacteria are linked to leanness and certain types linked to obesity. It seems that eating a particular diet (such as the modern Western one) can predispose those with bacteria linked to obesity to becoming obese. However adjusting the diet to reflect that of more traditional cultures can lend itself towards a leaner individual. Also a lack of the bacteria that help us to maintain a steady weight, brought about by antibiotic use, is linked to obesity. Identifying a specific blend of probiotics that could help weight reduction is not far off.

Chapter 20

Are Prebiotics the New Probiotics?

What are prebiotics?

PREbiotics provide food for the bacteria already living in the gut whilst PRObiotics provide a direct infusion of bacteria that weren't there before. In general terms, prebiotics are formed of the fibre that good bacteria eat but that isn't digestible by humans. Prebiotics are easier to get from familiar foods than probiotics for which you might have to look at either supplementing or at a traditional kind of food called 'fermented food'.

Natural Sources of Prebiotics:		
Vegetables	**Fruits**	**Grains and Legumes**
Asparagus	Apples	Beans
Chicory Root	Bananas	Chia seeds
Cabbage	Berries	Chickpeas
Fennel	Kiwis	Flaxseeds
Garlic		Green Peas
Jerusalem Artichoke		Lentils
Onions		Oats
Leeks		Quinoa
Pak Choi		

What about resistant starch?

It is important, in this section, also to note how resistant starch can play an important part in providing the fuel for probiotic bacteria. Although we used to think that starch was fully digested and absorbed in the small intestine, we now know that this is not the case. Resistant starch is the starch which is not digested, and is absorbed as glucose, in the small intestine. So it reaches the large intestine intact where all those microbes can get to work to convert it into very useful short chain fatty acids, such as butyrate. You can think of resistant starch like a fermentable fibre. In fact, resistant starch could soon be classified as a prebiotic too.

Resistant Starch – Dietary Sources:
Cooked and cooled potatoes
Cooked and cooled rice
Cooked and cooled legumes
Underripe plantains
Green (unripe) bananas
Plantain Flour
Teff Flour
Tapioca Flour
Potato Starch (not potato flour)

Therefore, how a food is prepared can determine how much resistant starch it will contain. Cooking and cooling certain foods means the starch remains resistant. Whilst eating it hot may be a missed opportunity for good bacteria to thrive.

How should you introduce prebiotics and resistant starch?
If you are unused to these foods in your diet or have digestive issues you should introduce them very slowly. Small amounts should be introduced at first and then you can gradually build up the amount that you consume over time. If too much is introduced too soon, digestive issues may result.

Should you buy probiotic supplements with prebiotics in them?
Although prebiotics are derived from food predominantly, increasingly, manufacturers of probiotics are throwing prebiotics into the same supplement and selling the supplement as a combined solution. Prebiotics have been shown to enhance the effectiveness of probiotics. However they're not all good news if supplemented in this way. Of particular concern is the prebiotic known as inulin. Inulin can serve as a food source to pathogens too. There is evidence to suggest that inulin can be broken down in the gastrointestinal tract by pathogens such as Klebsiella, and can serve as an energy source for pathogenic bacteria like Escherichia coli, Clostridium species and even certain yeasts. It has also been shown that pathogenic bacteria and yeasts might adapt and adopt prebiotics as a food source. When that happens, prebiotics will not selectively promote the growth of probiotics. Rather, prebiotics will fuel the spread of highly competitive pathogens and their dominance in the gut flora.

The role of prebiotics as a fuel source for yeast overgrowth and the replication of harmful bacteria is important because more manufacturers are adding prebiotics to probiotic products. The most common prebiotic added to probiotic products is FOS or fructooligosaccharides. This is extracted from natural sources and used in high concentrations in probiotics as an alternative sweetener and a microbial food source. Common side effects of FOS include wind, bloating, diarrhoea, abdominal pain and cramps. These are due to the release of gas from the breakdown of prebiotics by the bacteria living in the large intestine.

However, the potential to also promote the growth of pathogens in the gut means you should be cautious when choosing probiotics fortified with prebiotics. If you experience any adverse side effects when taking a combined prebiotic and probiotic supplement you may wish to take probiotics without prebiotics in and choose to introduce prebiotics in food form instead. If you cannot find prebiotic free probiotics where you live, you can take your probiotics in the form of fermented foods and eat real food sources of prebiotics and resistant starch, introducing both slowly.

In summary, whilst we can all benefit from the addition of prebiotics and resistant starch in our diet we should do so via natural food sources predominantly. We may choose to use a combined prebiotic and probiotic supplement but must monitor our reactions to this combination. Both prebiotic and probiotic food sources should be introduced slowly so as not to cause digestive problems. Food sources of prebiotics and resistant starch are abundant in a real food diet.

Chapter 21

Which Foods and Drinks Contain Probiotics?

There are many foods and drinks that are naturally rich in probiotics. Most often, probiotics are created via fermentation. Friendly bacteria are all around us so fermentation simply collects them and gives them a nice place to grow. Fermentation organisms produce alcohol, lactic acid, and acetic acid, preservatives that retain nutrients and prevent spoilage.

Probiotics are found in yogurt, buttermilk, kefir, sauerkraut, kimchi, and bacterially cultured cheese among other foods. Traditional methods of meat preservation (such as the curing of salami) also use fermentation of lactobacilli to preserve the food, although arguably industrially produced cured meats no longer have these health benefits.

Fermentation has a long history

When people talk about probiotics they often refer to substances added to food or indeed to food supplements. However, despite the fact that the word probiotic was not used until the twentieth century, many historic cultures used fermented food as a cheap way of preserving goods to be eaten out of season. This practice goes back thousands of years, and is still used in some parts of the world today. Earliest recordings of fermenting food date back to 6000 BC, where it was common in parts of the Middle East. The Romans used to eat sauerkraut for both its taste and its health benefits. Since then, nearly every civilisation has included fermented foods in their diet. Just think about German sourdough pretzels, traditionally pickled gherkins or the salamis and preserved olives from Italy. Some of the more traditional fermented foods are now becoming popular in parts of the world, areas where they've not been traditionally used. Examples include kimchi, kefir, kombucha, and sauerkraut, and even traditionally made yogurts and cheeses could be considered to be fermented. However, the probiotic value is compromised by modern processing methods which is why it's important to choose the source of your fermented foods carefully or indeed to make your own.

Traditional fermented foods

The recent resurgence and increased global popularity of fermented foods has inspired us to look at the way more traditional, cultures have managed to craft unique flavours around fermentation according to the availability of raw ingredients in their locations. Globally, there's quite a history of preserving foods and many of these methods have survived into modern times and are now being adopted across the world. In the table below, you'll find familiar names that are now popping up on the menus of restaurants, in continental stores and even in shops selling 'on-the-run' foods at service stations and transport hubs.

These fermented foods originated in:	
Japan – various forms of fermented soy	Natto Tempeh Tofu Miso Tamari
China	Douchi (black beans) Kombucha (tea)
Thailand	Nam Pla (fish sauce)
Korea	Kimchi (cabbage)
Ukraine	Raw yogurt Sauerkraut (cabbage) Buttermilk
Bulgaria	Kefir (cultured milk)
India	Lassi (yogurt drink)
Germany	Sauerkraut (cabbage) Sourdough Bread
Russia	Kefir

What does fermentation do?

Fermentation not only boosts good bacteria levels but also helps to eliminate anti-nutrients. It also means that:

1. The food is more digestible
2. The food has more minerals as there are less nutrient-binding phytates
3. The food has more protein as more protein is broken down by enzymes, making it more bioavailable
4. The food contains Vitamin B12 as a product of bacterial fermentation. Fermentation can create a reliable form of this nutrient which is often devoid in the diets of vegans.

Foods naturally fermented

Some foods that are naturally fermented have been around for years and are very simple to use:

- Tea - Most tea is fermented. Fermentation intensifies the stimulant properties of the leaves and produces the black and oolong varieties. Green tea is unfermented but does offer other nutritional benefits

- Sourdough bread - Sourdough is made from a combination of wild yeast and lactobacillus bacteria that are left to thrive and multiply in flour and water. The yeast and bacteria form a symbiotic relationship whereby the lactobacillus bacteria consume starches in the flour and create lactic acid. This is the most traditional form of bread production and it is the process still used in traditional bakeries in many parts of the world, and also now, in some artisan bakeries in the UK. Obviously bread must be baked and the high heat will render the live bacteria inert. However the benefits of the fermentation process leave you with bread that is:
  - Lower in glycaemic index i.e. it releases sugar into the bloodstream far more slowly than 'normal' bread.
  - More digestible:
    - As the starches have been predigested by bacteria in the early stages of fermentation, it is easier for humans to digest too.
    - The gluten in the bread is also more digestible.

- Cheese - Cheese is made using starter bacteria, but during the ripening process other (mainly lactic acid), bacteria grow spontaneously. These are often probiotic bacteria and are thought to arrive either via the milk or often through specific ingredients used by particular cheese producers. Bifidobacteria survives well in some Cheddar and Gouda cheese.[165] Hard and semi-hard Scandinavian cheeses tend to grow L paracasei predominantly as well as other lactobacillus strains.[166] Cheddars have been found with growth of L. casei, L. plantarum and L.brevis. Recent studies are finding that Propionibacterium which is used to make Emmental cheese may also have probiotic qualities. As with all products containing living bacteria, probiotic products must be cooled during storage. If heated, they won't survive. So cheeses must be unpasteurised (raw) to be able to offer their probiotic benefits.

- Yogurt – Yogurt is made from fermentation of the lactose in milk by L. delbrueckii subsp. Bulgaricus. This results in lactic acid which acts on milk protein to give yoghurt its texture and its characteristic acidic taste. There are other bacteria found in yoghurt including L. acidophilus, L. casei, Streptococcus salivarius subsp. thermophilus and Bifidobacterium Bifidus.

Fermentation can prevent food poisoning

In addition to supporting human health, lactobacillus and other bacteria may also protect against foodborne illness by inhibiting and eradicating foodborne pathogens, including Listeria monocytogenes, Staphylococcus aureus and Bacillus cereus. The inhibition of pathogenic bacteria may be due in part to the pH of the bacteria and their products, as well as antimicrobial properties produced by the probiotic bacteria that effectively compete with the unwanted microbes.

Fermentation has been used as a method of making foods safe to eat for years in several cultures. In West African countries, cassava or tapioca is an important food source. It contains natural cyanides and, if not properly fermented, can be poisonous to humans. In Scandinavia, fermentation is used to prevent raw fish from rotting. Fermented milk drinks, consumed worldwide, help increase the longevity or shelf-life of the milk whilst also improving digestibility.

Small batches vs. large-scale production

Traditional lacto-fermentation uses the bacteria naturally present on vegetables and a lactic acid bacteria starter culture. Once upon a time, all pickles were naturally fermented through lacto-fermentation, which is why some people use the terms 'pickled' and 'fermented' interchangeably. In modern times, this is no longer the case.

In large-scale 'pickled' food manufacturing, vegetables are washed in diluted chlorine solutions to destroy or inactivate bacteria. Acetic acid (which, along with water, is a main component of vinegar) is used instead of lactic acid. There are some commercially available pickles that are lacto-fermented but many are heat-treated or pasteurised to create a sterile product. Others are 'desalted' or rinsed, removing any beneficial bacteria that may have been present.

If it is health benefits that you are after, lacto-fermented foods work best from both quality and food safety perspectives when produced in small batches, and there are some small-scale operations that pride themselves on reinvigorating the fermented food market (look for them at gourmet stores, farmers markets and Asian shops). Meanwhile, home fermentation enthusiasts continue to grow in number. Home produced fermented foods are much cheaper to produce than to buy after some initial investment. However, one way to approach this is to try some of the shop bought products, see what suits you and your health objectives, then plan to make your own version at home.

Shop-Bought Probiotic Foods:
Kefir
Raw Apple Cider Vinegar
Roquefort
Sauerkraut
Kombucha
Kimchi
Fermented Miso
Sourdough
Cultured Vegetables

Make your own

The opportunities are numerous when it comes to making your own fermented foods. Vegetables such as cabbages, carrots, garlic, olives, cucumbers, onions, turnips, radishes, cauliflower and peppers, as well as multiple fruits such as lemons or berries, lend themselves to fermentation. The options are so wide that fermentation is becoming an increasingly popular part of people's lives. Lactic acid fermentation, or lacto-fermentation, is one of the most common methods and one of the easiest to experiment with at home. It is an anaerobic process whereby lactic acid bacteria, mainly lactobacillus species, convert sugar into lactic acid, which acts as a preservative. Salt plays a pivotal role in traditional fermentation by creating conditions that favour the bacteria, preventing the growth of pathogenic microorganisms, pulling water and nutrients from the food and adding flavour.

In conclusion, the market for fermented foods, in countries where traditional fermentation processes have been long forgotten, has never been larger. In fact, in 2016, kefir sales grew by sixteen per cent and kombucha sales by seven per cent across Europe[167]. Whilst many food cultures have been preparing fermented food and drink for millennia, those in other cultures are just catching on and are starting to adopt these traditional methods. They are doing so in order to achieve the health benefits that more traditional fermenting cultures have known about for years. Gut health can be rebalanced using a combination of probiotics in food or supplement form or both, plus prebiotics and resistant starch. Combinations of these traditional foods, displacing modern processed alternatives, are now being used to address many modern Western ailments from high cholesterol, through to IBS and mental health. However, typically, these are not prescribed by medics and rather it is being left to the individual to make the right choices about which combinations are best for them.

Chapter 22

Boosting the Immune System starting with the Gut

We have discovered that Hippocrates was not far wrong when he said, 'all disease begins in the gut.' This being the case, it is important to try and restore the health of the gut. This can have major positive effects on your entire body from your mood, to your weight and your vulnerability to disease. In fact, world renowned paediatric gastroenterologist Allesio Fasano, MD goes as far as to say:

> *The intestinal barrier operates as the biological door to inflammation, autoimmunity and cancer'*

How to improve your gut health:

Get to the root cause. While there can be many contributory factors for gut troubles it's always worth trying to identify the root cause before you attempt to mask the symptoms with medication. First of all run through this checklist:

1. Do you filter your water?
2. Do you avoid antibiotics, steroids medication and hormones as far as possible?
3. Do you choose food and drink carefully when travelling? Do you avoid raw and potentially contaminated food and drink bottled water?
4. Do you avoid mould exposure in your work or home environment?
5. Does your diet contain a range of natural foods including prebiotic and probiotic foods?
6. Do you have a significant amount of stress in your life?
7. Do you sleep well at night? i.e. do you have a regular circadian rhythm?
8. Were you born by C-section? Were you breast-fed? Was your mother's diet a healthy one?

Overhaul your diet. This is not something that should be undertaken lightly as there can be major side effects and withdrawal symptoms associated with dietary changes. Your new diet should aim to vastly reduce or eliminate sugar and refined carbohydrate foods. This approach can have a positive effect on the microbiome. The next step is the introduction of prebiotic rich foods and resistant starches with a continued supplementation of probiotics and/or fermented foods such as sauerkraut, kefir and kombucha to repopulate the gut with beneficial bacteria.

Eliminate problem foods. Foods that are beneficial for some people might not be good for you. If you are having digestive problems, then take a look at how some of the foods you may be eating could be causing your issues to worsen. These are only a problem for some people, not all.

- Lectins: particular types of proteins. The most irritating type is found in foods such as grains, beans, legumes, and nuts.
- Gluten and other similar proteins (such as hordein in barley, secalin in rye, or zein in corn), found in grains.
- Casein and/or lactose in dairy.
- Fructose (aka fruit sugar). People who struggle to digest fructose also often have trouble with other carbohydrates known as FODMAPs (fermentable oligosaccharides, disaccharides, monosaccharides and polyols).

Foods to avoid for a low FODMAP diet.

FODMAP	Foods to avoid
Fructose	• *Fruits:* apples, boysenberries, cherries (>3), figs, pears, nashi pears, peaches, mango, watermelon, tamarillo, tinned fruit, dried fruit, large serves of fruit • *Vegetables:* asparagus, arthichokes, sugar snap peas • *Sweeteners:* honey, frutose (>5g daily*), high fructose corn syrup • *Drinks:* fruit juice, soft drinks sweetened with fructose, sparkling wine, dessert wine, ciders, rum
Fructans	• *Fruits:* custard apples, nectarines, peaches, persimmon, rambutan, tamarillo, watermelon • *Vegetables:* artichokes, asparagus (>3), beetroot (>4 slices), Brussel sprouts (>½ cup), broccoli (>½ cup), cabbage-savoy (> 1cup), chicory root, corn (>½ cob), fennel (½ cup), garlic, leeks, okra, onions, peas (⅓ cup), radicchio lettuce, snow peas (>10), spring onion (white part) • *Cereals:* wheat, rye, barley products (bread, pasta, couscous, crackers, biscuits) • *Nuts:* cashews, pistachios
Galactans	• *Legumes:* all (chickpeas, lentils, dried/canned beans, baked beans, soy beans) • *Drinks:* soy milk
Lactose	• *Milk:* cow, goat and sheep • *Cheese:* fresh (cottage, ricotta, cream cheese, mascarpone) • *Other diary products:* yoghurt, ice cream, custard

FODMAP	Foods to avoid
Polyols	• *Fruits:* apples, apricots, avocado (>¼), blackberries, cherries (>3), longan (>10), lychees (>5), nashi pears, nectarines, pears, peaches, plums, prunes, watermelon • *Vegetables:* caulliflower, celery (>1 stick), mushrooms, snow peas, sweet potato (>½ cup) • *Sweeteners:* sorbitol (420), mannitol (421), xylitol (967), maltitol (965), isomalt (953)
	*up to 5g daily of fructose may be consumed if taken with meals

For some, certain compounds in foods can trigger mast cells to produce histamine, mimicking a food allergy and increasing intestinal permeability (leaky gut) and inflammation. The immune system can also start a reaction that manifests as respiratory allergies, such as sneezing, sniffles, and throat irritation. For others, these foods stimulate an immune system T-cell response and create or exacerbate autoimmune symptoms such as joint pain or skin rashes (particularly eczema). Some people simply lack the appropriate digestive enzymes to process one or more of these compounds. In this case, they might just feel a general stomach upset, gas and bloating, nausea, and constipation or diarrhoea. It is therefore important to identify these foods and eliminate those that may be causing you to react.

See: Overhaul Your Diet above.

Eat when hungry, stop when satisfied. Gut problems are often related to overconsumption of sugars, processed grains, processed meats, dairy, and rich meals. Try to eat meals based on good quality proteins and a range of brightly coloured vegetables as well as some lower sugar fruits such as berries, stone fruits and grapefruit. Eating real food meals makes it far easier to stop when you are satisfied and not to overeat.

Eat Mindfully
A simple checklist to follow when eating is:

SEEING - What does the food I am eating look like? Think about its colour, size and shape.
FEELING - What does it feel like? Is it hard, meltingly soft, crunchy?
SMELLING - Is it sweet, sour, aromatic?
THOUGHTS - What are your thoughts about this food? Positive or negative?
EMOTIONS - How are you feeling as you eat it? Do you like it? Does it remind you of something or somewhere from your past?

Slow down. The process of slowing down and chewing is important for acid production and enzyme release and breaking food down into particles that are manageable for the gut. Remember that the process of digestion begins when we even smell and see food. This is a reminder that preparing our own foods can improve the effectiveness of our digestive system.

Supplement wisely. There are many supplements that support your digestive health, but I believe the most beneficial leaky gut supplements are probiotics, l-glutamine, digestive enzymes, quercetin, and liquorice root. Both Sacchromyces Boulardii and glutathione may also be helpful in bringing about improvements to gut health.

Probiotics – Probiotics are the most important supplement or food to take. In short, they help to replenish good bacteria and crowd out bad bacteria. I recommend getting probiotics in both food and supplement form. Look at probiotics as a way of re-inoculating your gut with beneficial bacteria that will keep bad bacteria at bay.

L-Glutamine – L-Glutamine powder is an essential amino acid supplement that is anti-inflammatory and necessary for the growth and repair of your intestinal lining. Glutamine can therefore help reverse excessive intestinal permeability, act as fuel for intestinal cells, and might even reduce the severity of allergic reactions.

Digestive enzyme supplements. Choose a broad-based multi-enzyme formula but also consider betaine hydrochloride (HCl) as an addition. As we age, many of us produce less hydrochloric acid (stomach acid) so look for a digestive enzyme formula that includes betaine HCl on the label. However, if this combined formula gives you discomfort then keep to an enzyme supplement without betaine HCl. Using digestive enzymes decreases the chance that partially digested food particles and proteins are damaging your gut wall.

Quercetin – Quercetin is a plant flavonoid with strong antioxidant properties. It has also been shown to improve gut barrier function by sealing the gut because it supports the formation of proteins that help to keep the cells of the gut lining tightly together. It also stabilises mast cells and reduces the release of histamine, which is common in food intolerance. Taken before eating, it may block reactions to intolerant foods which might otherwise worsen symptoms of a leaky gut.

Liquorice Root – Liquorice is a herb that helps balance levels of the hormone cortisol (related to the management of stress and reduction of inflammation) and improves acid production in the stomach. It supports the body's natural processes for maintaining a healthy and intact stomach lining. This herb is especially beneficial for anyone who suffers from leaky gut brought about by emotional stress.

Sacchromyces Boulardii - Depending on the cause of the leaky gut, this specific yeast which is non-pathogenic should be considered. It has been widely used in Europe to treat diarrhoea. In France, it is popularly called 'yeast against yeast', and is thought to help clear the skin as well as the gut. Studies[168] have revealed the effectiveness for S. boulardii in the treatment or prevention of C. difficile diarrhoea, antibiotic diarrhoea and traveller's diarrhoea.

Glutathione (GSH) - Low levels of liver GSH tend to be found in those suffering from leaky gut, and it is an important part of your immune defence against tissue damage. It's an antioxidant that can eat up those free radicals that might otherwise be causing damage to the lining of your gut. The best way to raise GSH levels is to supplement cysteine or methionine which both convert to GSH in the body.

Check vitamin D levels - Vitamin D should be thought of more as a hormone in terms of its function than a vitamin. There are receptors for vitamin D in our entire gastrointestinal tract. We make vitamin D as a result of sun exposure mostly, but a lack of sun in many areas of the world and modern social practices mean lots of people are vitamin D deficient. According to the British government, a quarter of people have low vitamin D levels. The vitamin D we make on our skin goes to the liver, then into the bile that we need to break down fats. Low levels are associated with poor stomach emptying as well as bloating and poor bowel movements. A possible explanation for this is that if we do not supply our gut with sufficient Vitamin D then the good gut bacteria can die off. In turn, this can be linked to Vitamin B deficiency.

Support vitamin B levels - Gut bacteria helps manufacture vitamins, especially B vitamins. Vitamin B5 and B12 are crucial for energy and sleep balance. As we found out earlier in this book, energy levels and poor sleep can affect the gut bacteria so supplementing or eating foods rich in B vitamins could help get your gut bacteria back on the right track again. B vitamins can be found in green vegetables, potatoes, wholegrains, some cheese – remember unpasteurised cheeses are more likely to contain probiotics too - eggs, yogurt, poultry, nuts, seeds, legumes, and mushrooms.

Check iron levels - Decreased iron status is associated with poor gut function. This can be caused by poor absorption of iron, or simply insufficient consumption of iron rich foods. Remember that vitamin C foods can increase the rate of absorption of iron so aim to eat both sources of food together. Ideal combinations include sardines with salad, apple wedges with almond butter and steak with spinach, broccoli and tomatoes.

Get the right fats - While consumption of vegetable oils is known to increase the free radicals in the body and therefore inflammation, eating the right fats has been shown to reduce this. Eating plenty of Omega 3s (flax, walnuts, hemp, chia, fish, algae such as chlorella and spirulina) and other whole food fats (olives, avocado, coconut, nuts, seeds) can help moderate inflammation. Particular saturated fats are also healthy when it comes to intestinal health. Butter, for example, contains a fatty acid called butyrate that helps heal the gut lining and reduce inflammation. Lauric acid, a fat found in coconut oil, is also thought to improve gut health. Not only is this fat easy to digest it is now being studied for its antifungal, antiviral and antibacterial properties.

Flavonoids can help improve gut health - Gut bacteria and the flavonoids found in vegetables and fruits predominantly exist in a two way relationship. Whilst the flavonoids tend to arrive in the large intestine intact and serve as fuel for the trillions of bacteria there, it appears that flavonoids can also have a positive effect on gut bacterial balance as they can help to change it for the better. Of course, a diet that incorporates a range of colourful vegetables and fruit is a healthy one for most people but foods to focus on in particular are leeks, cabbage, Brussels sprouts, and vegetable broths. If you are struggling to digest these foods, then aim for a range of brightly coloured vegetables and fruit in your diet on a daily basis.

Recover well - Sleep, stress management and exercise are necessary for renewing calls and maintaining the integrity of the gut lining as well as for keeping inflammation in check. Improving these areas can also improve gut health. Try to stick to routines, take regular breaks from work and incorporate enjoyable and sustainable exercise into your week.

Just eat real food - Our bodies have a strong and longstanding relationship with real food. Food preservatives and additives, the kind you find in processed foods, present a new (and perhaps impossible) challenge for our bodies. Michael Pollan is a well-known food author has said that we should eat food not edible food-like substances. Try to find foods with recognisable ingredients that have a clear origin. For example, blueberries and Greek yogurt are far more easily recognised and digested by your body than a blueberry flavoured yogurt.

Get fibre - Nutrient dense, high-fibre carbohydrates like vegetables are an important part of a healthy diet. Try to consume fibre in the form of real foods. Add more vegetables, fruit, nuts, seeds, beans, peas, and wholegrains to your diet.

Breastfeed - Children who are breastfed tend to have less gastrointestinal infections and inflammatory disorders so it makes sense, where feasible, to breastfeed for at least six months.

Expose children to germs - Being exposed to lots of germs in childhood seems to be linked to a reduced incidence of atopic diseases such as asthma and eczema, which we have already discovered are often linked to poor gut health. It seems that the more exposure children have to bugs in their environment when young, the more immunity they build up and the stronger their gut becomes as an immune defence mechanism.

Expose mums to probiotics - If you are expecting a baby and a C-section is likely, then research suggests that the likely reduction in bifidobactrium due to birthing method could be improved with supplementation of prebiotics and the probiotic bifidobacterium animalis subsp. Lactis.[169]

Reduce the chemical burden on your body - Choose organic food when possible, avoid heating foods in plastics and the use of vegetable oils. Think about the products you use on your skin and your face. Try to avoid food colorings, preservatives, emulsifiers, artificial sweeteners and unnecessary drugs. Where possible, try to find alternative treatments to using NSAIDs (such as ibuprofen), acid blockers, and antibiotics because, as we have discovered, these harm our healthy bacteria, disrupt the delicate chemical ecosystem of our GI tracts, and cause additional gut damage.

Poop when your body tells you to - This seems like a simple thing but so many people hold off pooping when they really need to go. If you need to go, then you should, because withholding can cause your stools to dry out and become harder to pass.

As we look towards the future we must understand that improving gut health is an investment in our long-term health. Further research into the microbiome will identify the multitude of ways in which probiotics, prebiotics and resistant starch could be used in creating better health outcomes. Further research would undoubtedly also refine the way in which the medical world predict, prevent, diagnose and treat ill-health in the future too.

Notes

CHAPTER 1

1 O' Keefe S.J. et al, 'Fat, fibre and cancer risk in African Americans and rural Africans', Nature Communication, vol.6 (2015) , p6342

2 Wilson, Claire. "Parkinson's Disease May Start In The Gut And Travel To The Brain". New Scientist 2016

3 Bravo, J.A, 'Ingestion of Lactobacillus strain regulates emotional behavior and central GABA receptor expression in a mouse via the vagus nerve', Proceedings of the National Academy of Sciences, vol 108, pp16050-16055

4 Schmidt, K. et al, 'P.1.e.003 Prebiotic intake reduces the waking cortisol response and alters emotional bias in healthy volunteers', European Neuropsychopharmacology, vol. 24, pp S191

5 Wilson, Claire. "Parkinson's Disease May Start In The Gut And Travel To The Brain". New Scientist 2016

6 Challis, C. '468.15 / NNN5 - Progression of Parkinson's-like pathology following inoculation of alpha-synuclein preformed fibrils in the gut', 468 - Optical Methods: Probe Development and Applications (2016)

7 Kostic, A.D et al, 'The Dynamics of the Human Infant Gut Microbiome in Development and in Progression toward Type 1 Diabetes', Cell Host and Microbiome, vol.17 (2016), pp260-273

8 Paun, A. 'Modulation of type 1 and type 2 diabetes risk by the intestinal microbiome', Pediatric Diabetes, vol 17 (2016), pp469-477

CHAPTER 3

9 Gosalbes M,J. Meconium microbiota types dominated by lactic acid or enteric bacteria are differentially associated with maternal eczema and respiratory problems in infants. Clinical & Experimental Allergy, vol. 43 (2013), pp198-211

10 Jakobsson, H, E. Decreased gut microbiota diversity, delayed Bacteroidetes colonisation and reduced Th1 responses in infants delivered by Caesarean section. Gut, vol.63 (2013), pp- 559-566

11 Bainbridge, J. Breast milk boosts growth of beneficial gut flora. British Journal of Midwifery. Vol. 20 (2012), pp 821-821

12 Everard, A. Cross-talk between Akkermansia muciniphila and intestinal epithelium controls diet-induced obesity. PNAS. Vol. 110 (2013) pp 9066–9071

13 Wang, K. Development of a real-time PCR method for Firmicutes and Bacteroidetes in faeces and its application to quantify intestinal population of obese and lean pigs. Letters in Applied Microbiology, vol.47 (2008), pp 367-373

14 Rastmanesh, R. High polyphenol, low probiotic diet for weight loss because of intestinal microbiota interaction. Chemico-Biological Interactions, vol. 189 (2011), pp1-8

15 Christoph A, T. et al. Transkingdom Control of Microbiota Diurnal Oscillations Promotes Metabolic Homeostasis. Cell. Vol. 159 (3) (2014) pp514-529

16 Penders, J. et al. Factors influencing the composition of the intestinal microbiota in early infancy. Pediatrics, vol. 118 (2) (2006) pp 511-521

CHAPTER 4

17 Deng, K. et al. In vitro and in vivo examination of anticolonization of pathogens by Lactobacillus paracasei FJ861111.1. Journal of Dairy Science, vol.98 (10) (2015), pp 6759-66

18 Kovachev, S. Probiotic monotherapy of bacterial vaginosis: an open, randomized trial. Akusherstro i Ginekologiyz, vol. 52 (2013), pp 36-42

19 Ortiz-Lucas, M. et al. Effect of probiotic species on irritable bowel syndrome symptoms: A bring up to date meta-analysis. Revista Española de Enfermedades Digestiva, vol. 105 (1) (2013), pp 19-36

20 Nobaek, S. et al. Alteration of intestinal microflora is associated with reductions in abdominal bloating and pain in patients with irritable bowel syndrome. The American Journal of Gastroenterology, vol. 95(5) (2000), pp 1231-1238

21 Niedzielin, K. A controlled, double-blind, randomized study on the efficacy of Lactobacillus plantarum 299V in patients with irritable bowel syndrome. European Journal of Gastroenterology & Hepatology, vol. 13(10) (2001), pp 1143-1147.

22 Pakdaman M, N. et al. The effects of the DDS-1 strain of lactobacillus on symptomatic relief for lactose intolerance - a randomized, double-blind, placebo-controlled, crossover clinical trial. Nutrition Journal, vol.15 (1) (2015).

23 Fabbrocini, G. et al. Supplementation with Lactobacillus rhamnosus SP1 normalises skin expression of genes implicated in insulin signalling and improves adult acne. Beneficial Microbes, vol. 7 (5) (2016), pp 625-630

24 Martoni, C. J and Prakash, S. Daily doses of a new probiotic reduces 'bad' and total cholesterol. American Heart Association. November 05, 2012

25 DiRienzo D. B. Effect of probiotics on biomarkers of cardiovascular disease: implications for heart-healthy diets. Nutrition Reviews, vol. 72 (1) (2013) pp 18-29

26 Mikelsaar, M. Lactobacillus fermentum ME-3 - an antimicrobial and antioxidative probiotic. Microbial Ecology in Health & Disease, vol. 21 (1) (2009)

27 Yazdi, M. et al. Selenium nanoparticle-enriched Lactobacillus brevis causes more efficient immune responses in vivo and reduces the liver metastasis in metastatic form of mouse breast cancer. DARU Journal of Pharmaceutical Sciences, vol. 21 (1) (2013), pp 33.

28 Della Riccia D, N. Anti-inflammatory effects of Lactobacillus brevis (CD2) on periodontal disease. Oral Disease, vol. 13 (4), pp376-385

29 Bendali, F. et al. Beneficial effects of a strain of Lactobacillus paracasei subsp. paracasei in Staphylococcus aureus-induced intestinal and colonic injury. International Journal of Infectious Diseases, vol.15 (11) (2011), pp e787-e794

30 Deguch, R et al. Effect of Pretreatment With Lactobacillus Gasseri OLL2716 on First-Line Helicobacter Pylori Eradication Therapy. J Gastroenterol Hepatol, vol. 27(5) (2012), pp 888-892.

31 Murri, M. et al. Gut microbiota in children with type 1 diabetes differs from that in healthy children: a case-control study. BOC Medicine, vol. 11 (1) (2013)

32 Kostic, A, D. et al. The Dynamics of the Human Infant Gut Microbiome in Development and in Progression toward Type 1 Diabetes. Cell Host & Microbe, vol. 20 (1) (2016), pp121

33 Yamano, T. et al. Effects of the probiotic strain Lactobacillus johnsonii strain La1 on autonomic nerves and blood glucose in rats. Life Sciences, vol. 79 (20) (2006), pp 1963-1967

34 Singh, S. et al. Lactobacillus rhamnosus NCDC17 ameliorates type-2 diabetes by improving gut function, oxidative stress and inflammation in high-fat-diet fed and streptozotocintreated rats. Beneficial Microbes, pp1-14

35 Qin, Z.R et al. Effect of Lactose and Lactobacillus acidophilus on the Colonization of Salmonella enteritidis in Chicks Concurrently Infected with Eimeria tenella. Avian Disease, vol. 39 (3) (1995), pp 548

36 Darby, B. et al. In vitro inhibition of growth of E. Coli, salmonella typhimurium, and clostridia perfringens using probiotics isolated from equine feces. March 16, 2015.

37 Avadhani A, Miley H. Probiotics for prevention of antibiotic-associated diarrhea and Clostridium difficile-associated disease in hospitalized adults: a meta-analysis. Journal of the American Academy of Nurse Practitioners, vol. 23 (6) (2011), pp269-274

38 Singh, T. P. et al. Antagonistic Activity of Lactobacillus reuteri Strains on the Adhesion Characteristics of Selected Pathogens. Frontiers in Microbiology, vol. 8 (2017)

39 Hiroshi, O. et al. Oral Administration Bifidobacterium bifidum G9-1 Suppresses Total and Antigen Specific Immunoglobulin E Production in Mice. Biological and Pharmaceutical Bulletin, vol. 28(8) pp 1462-1466

40 Schiavi, E. et al. Oral therapeutic administration of a probiotic mixture suppresses established Th2 responses and systemic anaphylaxis in a murine model of food allergy. Allergy vol. 66 (2011) pp 499–508.

41 Adel-Patient, K. et al. Oral administration of recombinant Lactococcus lactis expressing bovine beta-lactoglobulin partially prevents mice from sensitization. Clin Exp Allergy, vol.35 (2005); pp 539–546.

42 Cortes-Perez N,G. et al. Allergy therapy by intranasal administration with recombinant Lactococcus lactis producing bovine beta-lactoglobulin. Int Arch Allergy Immunol, vol 150 (2009), pp 25–31.

43 Martín, R. et al. The effects of selected probiotic strains on the development of eczema (the PandA study). Allergy, vol. 64(9) (2009), pp 1349-58.

44 Groeger, D. et al. Bifidobacterium infantis 35624 modulates host inflammatory processes beyond the gut. Gut Microbes, vol. 4(4) (2013), pp 325-339.

45 Collado M. et al. Imbalances in faecal and duodenal Bifidobacterium species composition in active and non-active coeliac disease. BMC Microbiology, vol. 8 (1) (2008), pp232

46 Lindfors, K. et al. Live probiotic Bifidobacterium lactis bacteria inhibit the toxic effects induced by wheat gliadin in epithelial cell culture. Clinical & Experimental Immunology, vol. 152 (3) (2008), pp 552-558

47 Yazawa, K. et al. Bifidobacterium longum as a delivery system for cancer gene therapy: Selective localization and growth in hypoxic tumors. Cancer Gene Therapy vol. 7 (2) (2000), pp 269–274.

48 Li, C et al. Selenium-Bifidobacterium longum as a delivery system of endostatin for inhibition of pathogenic bacteria and selective regression of solid tumor. Experimental and Therapeutic Medicine, vol. 1(1) (2010) pp 129-135.

49 Burton, J, P. et al. A preliminary study of the effect of probiotic Streptococcus salivarius K12 on oral malodour parameters.J Appl Microbiology, vol.100(4) (2006), pp754-764

CHAPTER 5

50 Arumugam, M. et al. Enterotypes of the human gut microbiome. Nature, vol. 473(7346) (2011), pp 174-180

51 Rojahn, R. et al. Journal Scan Wu GD , Chen J , Hoffman C (2011) Linking long-term dietary patterns with gut microbial enterotypes Science. Gastrointestinal Nursing, vol. 9 (8) (2011), pp 12

52 de Moraes A C et al. Enterotype May Drive the Dietary-Associated Cardiometabolic Risk Factors. Front Cell Infect Microbiol, vol. 23 (7), pp 47

53 Pop, M. et al. Diarrhea in young children from low-income countries leads to large-scale alterations in intestinal microbiota composition. Genome Biology, vol. 15 (6) (2014), pp R76

54 Moreno, J. et al. Prevotella copri and the microbial pathogenesis of rheumatoid arthritis. Reumatología Clínica (English Edition), vol. 11 (2) (2015), pp 61-63

55 Wang J. et al. Dietary history contributes to enterotype-like clustering and functional metagenomic content in the intestinal microbiome of wild mice. PNAS, vol. 111 (26) (2014), pp E2703–E2710

CHAPTER 6

56 Shorter R, G. et al. A working hypothesis for the etiology and pathogenesis of nonspecific inflammatory bowel disease. Digest Dis 1972

57 Lerner, A. et al. Transglutaminases in Dysbiosis As Potential Environmental Drivers of Autoimmunity. Frontiers In Microbiology, vol. 8 (2017)

58 Bailey, M. T. et al. Stressor Exposure Disrupts Commensal Microbial Populations in the Intestines and Leads to Increased Colonization by Citrobacter rodentium. Infection and Immunity, vol. 78 (4), (2010), pp 1509-1519

59 Bjarnason, I. et al. Metronidazole reduces intestinal inflammation and blood loss in non-steroidal anti-inflammatory drug induced enteropathy. Gut, vol. 33(9) (1992), pp 1204-8

60 Wilson, Claire. "Parkinson's Disease May Start In The Gut And Travel To The Brain". New Scientist 2016

CHAPTER 7

61 Suez, J. et al. Artificial Sweeteners Induce Glucose Intolerance by Altering the Gut Microbiota. Obstetrical & Gynecological Survey, vol. 70 (1) (2015), pp31-32

62 Giannela, R, A et al. Production of vitamin B12 analogues in patients with small bowel bacterial overgrowth. *Gastroenterology*, vol. 62(2) (1972), pp 255-60.

63 Dreyer, H, P, et al. Mucosal Permeation of Macromolecules and Particles, in Intestinal Absorption and Secretion. (1983); *MTP Press*; Hing Ham, pp 505-13.

64 Ionescu G. et al. Abnormal fecal microflora and malabsorption phenomena in atopic eczema patients. J Adv Med, vol. 3 (1990), p*p 71-89.*

65 Alun Jones V, et al. Food intolerance: a major factor in the pathogenesis of irritable bowel syndrome. Lancet, vol. 2 (1980), pp 1115-*1117.*

66 Hansen J, et al. The role of mucosal immunity and host genetics in defining intestinal commensal bacteria. Curr Opin Gastroenterol. vo*l. 26 (201), pp564–71.*

67 Beeken WL. Remedial defects in Crohn disease. Arch Int Med, vol.135 (1975), *pp 686-690.*

68 Hollander D, Vadheim C, Brettholz E, et al. Increased intestinal permeability in patients with Crohn's disease and their relatives. Ann Int Med, vol. 105 (1986), *pp 883-885*

69 Inman RD. Reactive arthritis, Reiter's syndrome, and enteric pathogens. Infections in The Rheumatic Diseases. In: Espinoza L, Goldenberg D, Arnett F, Alarcon G eds. Orlando, FL G*rune & Stratton; (1988) pp 273-280.*

70 Husby G, et al. Cross-reactive epitope with Klebslella pneumoniae nitrogenase in articular tissue of HLA-B27 + patients with ankylosing spondylitis. Arth Rheum, vol.32 (198*9), pp 437-445.*

CHAPTER 8

71 Vandeputte, D. et al. Stool consistency is strongly associated with gut microbiota richness and composition, enterotypes and bacterial growth rates. Gut, vol. 65(1) (2015), pp 57-62

CHAPTER 9

72 Prescott S, L . et al. Supplementation with Lactobacillus rhamnosus or Bifidobacterium lactis probiotics in pregnancy increases cord blood interferon-γ and breast milk transforming growth factor-γ and immunoglobin A detection. *Clinical & Experimental Allergy,* vol. 38 (10) (2008), pp 1606-1614

73 Rautava S et al. Maternal probiotic supplementation during pregnancy and breast-feeding reduces the risk of eczema in the infant. Journal of Allergy and Clinical Immunology, vol. 130 (6) (2012), pp1355-1360

74 Dachung Wu et al. ANTIOXIDANT PROPERTIES OF LACTOBACILLUS AND ITS PROTECTING EFFECTS TO OXIDATIVE STRESS CACO-2 CELLS. The Journal of Animal & Plant Sciences, vol. 24(6) (2014), pp1766-1771

75 Bernet M, et al. Lactobacillus acidophilus LA 1 binds to human intestinal cell lines and inhibits cell attachment and cell invasion by enterovirulent bacteria. *Gut,* vol.34 (1994), pp 483-9.

76 Pothoulakis C, et. al. Saccharomyces boulardii inhibits Clostridium difficile toxin A binding and enterotoxicity in rat ileum. *Gastroenterology* 104 (1993), pp 1108-15.

77 Malin M, et al. Promotion of IgA immune response in patients with Crohn's disease by oral bacteriotherapy with Lactobacillus GG. *Ann Nutr Metab*, vol. 40 (1996), pp137-45.

78 Silva M, et. al. Antimicrobial substance from a human Lactobacillus strain. *Antimicrob Agents Chemothe,* vol. 31 (1987), pp 1231-3.

79 Vandenbergh P. Lactic acid bacteria, their metabolic products and interference with microbial growth. *FEMS Microbiol Rev,* vol. 12 (1993), pp 221-38.

80 Salminen S. et al. Lactic acid bacteria in the gut in normal and disordered states. *Dig. Dis,* vol. 10 (1992), pp 227 – 38.

81 Oksanen P.J. et al. 1990. Prevention of traveller's diarrhea by Lactobacillus GG. *Ann. Med*, vol. 22, pp 53 – 56.

82 Isolauri E, et al. 1993. Lactobacillus casei strain GG reverses increased intestinal permeability induced by cows milk in suckling rats. *Gastroenterology*, vol.105, pp 643 – 1650.

83 Majamaa, H., E. Isolauri. Probiotics: A novel approach in the management of food allergy. *J. Allergy and Clin. Immunol.* (1997), pp 179 – 185

84 Maydannik V, Haytovich M, Sosnovska T & Kyrychenko I (2008) Prevention and treatment of antibiotic-associated diarrhoea. Paediatrics, Obstetrics & Gynaecology 1 63-65

85 Oliveira V, M. et al. Lactobacillus is able to alter the virulence and the sensitivity profile of Candida albicans. J Appl Microbiology, vol. 121(6) *(2016), pp 1737-1744*

86 Murakami, T. et al (2006) Safety and effect of yoghurt containing Bifidobacterium lactis BB-12® on improvement of defecation and faecal microflora in healthy volunteers. Journal of Nutritional *Food, vol. 9, pp. 15-26*

87 Uchida et al. (2005) Effect of fermented milk containing Bifidobacterium lactis BB-12® on stool frequency, defecation, fecal microbiota and safety of excessive ingestion in healthy female students. Jou*rnal of Nutritional Food, vol. 8(1) (2005), pp.39-51*

88 Macfarland, L. Meta-analysis of probiotics for the prevention of traveller's diarrhea. Travel Medicine and Inf*ectious Disease, vol. 5 (2) pp 97-105*

89 UK One Health Report Joint report on human and animal antibiotic use, sales and resistance, 2013. (2018).

CHAPTER 10

90 UK One Health Report Joint report on human and animal antibiotic use, sales and resistance, 2013

91 Schaumburg, I. Could probiotics be the next big thing in acne and rosacea treatments? *American Academy of* Dermatology (Feb. 3, 2014)

92 Schaumburg, I. Could probiotics be the next big thing in acne and rosacea treatments? *American Academy of* Dermatology (Feb. 3, 2014)

93 Cochrane Library. Probiotics for persistent diarrhoea in children. *Cochrane Database of Systematic Reviews*. December 13, 2012.

94 Evans, M. et al. Effectiveness of Lactobacillus helveticus and Lactobacillus rhamnosus for the management of antibiotic-associated diarrhoea in healthy adults: a randomised, double-blind, placebo-controlled trial. *Br J Nutr*, vol. 116(1) (2016), pp94-103.

95 Anukam, K. et al. Augmentation of antimicrobial metronidazole therapy of bacterial vaginosis with oral probiotic Lactobacillus rhamnosus GR-1 and Lactobacillus reuteri RC-14: randomized, double-blind, placebo controlled trial. *Microbes Infect*, vol. 8(6) (2006), pp 1450-4.

96 http://modernhcp.com/video-how-should-we-be-taking-probiotics-in-relation-to-antibiotics/

CHAPTER 11

97 Rooney, P.J., R.T. Jenkins, and W.W. Buchanan, A short review of the relationship between intestinal permeability and inflammatory joint disease. Clin Exp Rheumatol, 1990. 8(1): p. 75-83

98 Katz, K.D., et al., Intestinal permeability in patients with Crohn's disease and their healthy relatives. Gastroenterology, 1989. 97*(4): p. 927-31.*

99 Munkholm, P., et al., Intestinal permeability in patients with Crohn's disease and ulcerative colitis and their first degree relatives. Gut, 1994. 35(1): p. 68-72.

100 Pearson, A.D., et al., Intestinal permeability in children with Crohn's disease and coeliac disease. Br Med J, 1982. 285(6334): p. 20-1.

101 Hamilton, I., et al., Small intestinal permeability in dermatological disease. Q J Med, 1985. 56(221): p. 559-67.

102 Tepper, R.E., et al., Intestinal permeability in patients infected with human immunodeficiency virus. Am J Gastroenterol, 1994. 89: p. 878-882.

103 Lewis J et al. Eliminating Immunologically-Reactive Foods from the Diet and its Effect on Body Composition and Quality of Life in Overweight Persons. *Journal Obesity & Weight loss Therapy*, vol. 2 (1) (2012)

104 https://en.wikipedia.org/wiki/Zonulin

CHAPTER 12

105 Zackular, P. et al. The Human Gut Microbiome as a Screening Tool for Colorectal Cancer. *Cancer Prevention Research.* (August 2014)

106 Lupascu A, et al. Hydrogen glucose breath test to detect small intestinal bacterial overgrowth: a prevalence case-control study in irritable bowel syndrome. *Aliment Pharmacol Ther*, vol. 22 (2005), pp 1157–1160.

107 Mann NS, Limoges-Gonzales M. The prevalence of small intestinal bacterial overgrowth in irritable bowel syndrome. *Hepatogastroenterology, vol.* 56 (2009), pp 718–721.

108 Rubio-Tapia A, et al. Prevalence of small intestine bacterial overgrowth diagnosed by quantitative culture of intestinal aspirate in celiac disease. *J Clin Gastroenterol*, vol. 43 (2009), pp 157–161.

109 Sabaté JM, et al. High prevalence of small intestinal bacterial overgrowth in patients with morbid obesity: a contributor to severe hepatic steatosis. *Obes Surg*, vol.18 (2008), pp 371–377.

110 Wyatt, J. et al. Intestinal permeability and the prediction of relapse in Crohn's disease. Lancet, vol. 341(8858) (1993) pp 1437-9.

111 De Boissieu, D et al. Allergy to nondairy proteins in mother's milk as assessed by intestinal permeability tests. *Revue Française d'Allergologie et d'Immunologie Clinique,* vol.35(4) (1995), pp 377-380

CHAPTER 13

112 McElhanon, B, O. et al. Gastrointestinal Symptoms in Autism Spectrum Disorder: A Meta-analysis. Pediatrics, April 2014

113 Gorrindo P, et al. Gastrointestinal dysfunction in autism: parental report, clinical evaluation, and associated factors. *Autism Research.* vol. 5(2), pp 101–108.

114 Song, Y. et al. Real-time PCR quantitation of clostridia in feces of autistic children. *Appl Environ Microbiol*, vol. 70(11) (2004), pp 6459-65.

115 ParrachoH, M. et al. Differences between the gut microflora of children with autistic spectrum disorders and that of healthy children. *J Med Microbiol.* Vol. 54(Pt 10) (2005), pp 987-91.

116 Gilbert, J, A, et al. Toward Effective Probiotics for Autism and Other Neurodevelopmental Disorders. Cell, vol. 155(7) (2013),pp1446–1448

117 Rosa Krajmalnik-Brown, Jin Gyoon; PLOS ONE, July 3rd, 2013

118 Wang, L. et al. Low Relative Abundances of the Mucolytic Bacterium Akkermansia muciniphila and Bifidobacterium spp. in Feces of Children with Autism. *Appl. Environ. Microbiol*, vol.77(18), pp 6718-6721

119 Owens, B. Gut microbe may fight obesity and diabetes. *Nature News,* May 13, 2013

120 https://www.theguardian.com/science/2006/sep/04/medicineandhealth. lifeandhealth

121 Wakefield, A. et al. RETRACTED: Ileal-lymphoid-nodular hyperplasia, non-specific colitis, and pervasive developmental disorder in children. The Lancet, vol. 351, (9103) (1998), pp637–641

122 Seekatz, A, M. et al. Differential Response of the Cynomolgus Macaque Gut Microbiota to Shigella Infection. *PLoS ONE*, vol. 8 (6) (2013), pp e64212

123 Eloe-Fadrosh, E, A. et al. Impact of Oral Typhoid Vaccination on the Human Gut Microbiota and Correlations with S. Typhi-Specific Immunological Responses. *PLoS ONE*, vol. 8 (4) (2013), pp e6202

124 Kandasamy, S. et al. Lactobacilli and Bifidobacteria enhance mucosal B cell responses and differentially modulate systemic antibody responses to an oral human rotavirus vaccine in a neonatal gnotobiotic pig disease model. *Gut Microbes*, vol. 5 (5) (2014)

125 Prharaj, S, et al. Probiotics, antibiotics and the immune responses to vaccines. Philosophical Transactions of the Royal Society B, vol. 370 (1671) (2015)

CHAPTER 14

126 Rhee, S, H. et al. Principles and clinical implications of the brain-gut-enteric microbiota axis. *Nat Rev Gastroenterol Hepatol*, vol. 6(5) (2009), pp306-14

127 Steenbergen, L. et al. A randomized controlled trial to test the effect of multispecies probiotics on cognitive reactivity to sad mood. *Brain, Behaviour and Immunity*, vol. 48 (2015), pp 258–264

128 http://newsroom.ucla.edu/releases/changing-gut-bacteria-through-245617

129 Bravo, J, A. et al. Ingestion of Lactobacillus strain regulates emotional behavior and central GABA receptor expression in a mouse via the vagus nerve. *Proc Natl Acad Sci* , vol. 108(38) (2011), pp 16050–16055.

130 Benton, D. et al. Impact of consuming a milk drink containing a probiotic on mood and cognition. *Eur J Clin Nutr, v*ol. 61(3) (2007), pp 355-61

131 Rao, A, V. et al. A randomized, double-blind, placebo-controlled pilot study of a probiotic in emotional symptoms of chronic fatigue syndrome. *Gut Pathog*. Vol. 1(1) (2006), pp 6.

132 Akbari, E. et al. The effects of probiotics on mental health and hypothalamic-pituitary-adrenal axis: A randomized, double-blind, placebo-controlled trial in petrochemical workers. *Front Aging Neurosc, vol.* 8 (256) (2016)

133 Rogers, G.B. et al. From gut dysbiosis to altered brain function and mental illness: mechanisms and pathways. *Mol Psychiatry*, vol. 21(6) (2016), pp 738-48

CHAPTER 15

134 www.rightdiagnosis.com

135 www.allergyuk.org

136 Penders, J. et al. Gut microbiota composition and development of atopic manifestations in infancy: the KOALA Birth Cohort Study. *Gut,* vol.56 (5)

137 Ciacci, C. et al. Allergy prevalence in adult celiac disease. *Journal of Allergy and Clinical Immunology*, vol.113(6), pp 1199–1203

138 Bonciolini, V. et al. Cutaneous Manifestations of Non-Celiac Gluten Sensitivity: Clinical Histological and Immunopathological Features. *Nutrients,* vol. 7(9) (2015), pp 7798–7805.

139 Isolauri,E. et al. Probiotics in the management of atopic eczema. Clinical & Experimental Allergy, vol.30 (2000), pp 1605–1610

140 Rosenfeldt, V. et al. Effect of probiotic Lactobacillus strains in children with atopic dermatitis. *Journal of Allergy and Clinical Immunology*, vol. 111(2) (2003), pp 389–395

141 Abrahamsson T,R,1. et al. Probiotics in prevention of IgE-associated eczema: a double-blind, randomized, placebo-controlled trial. *J Allergy Clin Immunol*, vol. 119(5) (2007), pp 1174-80

142 Kukkonen, K et al. Probiotics and prebiotic galacto-oligosaccharides in the prevention of allergic diseases: A randomized, double-blind, placebo-controlled trial . *Journal of Allergy and Clinical Immunology,* vol.119(1) (2007), pp 192-198

CHAPTER 16

143 Sudo, N. et al. The requirement of intestinal bacterial flora for the development of an IgE production system fully susceptible to oral tolerance induction. *J Immuno,* vol. 159(4) (1997), pp 739-45.

144 Schiavi, E. et al. Oral therapeutic administration of a probiotic mixture suppresses established Th2 responses and systemic anaphylaxis in a murine model of food allergy. *Allergy*, vol. 66 (2011), pp 499–508.

145 Stefka, A.T. et al. Commensal bacteria protect against food allergen sensitization. PNAS, vol. 111 (36) (2014), pp 13145–13150

146 Canani, R.B. et al. Effect of Lactobacillus GG on tolerance acquisition in infants with cow's milk allergy: a randomized trial. *J Allergy Clin Immunol*, vol. 129 (2012), pp 580–582.

147 Adel-Patient K, et al. Oral administration of recombinant Lactococcus lactis expressing bovine beta-lactoglobulin partially prevents mice from sensitization. *Clin Exp Allergy*, vol. 35 (2005), pp 539–546

148 Cortes-Perez N,G. et al. Allergy therapy by intranasal administration with recombinant Lactococcus lactis Producing bovine beta-lactoglobulin. *Int Arch Allergy Immunol, vol.* 150 (2009), pp 25–31

149 Huibregtse I, L. et al. Induction of ovalbumin-specific tolerance by oral administration of Lactococcus lactis secreting ovalbumin. *Gastroenterology*, vol. 133 (2207), pp 517–528.

CHAPTER 17

150 Mika, A. et al. Early life exercise may promote lasting brain and metabolic health through gut bacterial metabolites. *Immunology and Cell Biology*, vol. 94(2) (2015)

151 Choi, J, J. et al. Exercise Attenuates PCB-Induced Changes in the Mouse Gut Microbiome. Environ Health Perspect, vol.121(6) (2013)

152 Clarke, S et al. Exercise and associated dietary extremes impact on gut microbial diversity. Gut, vol.63(12) (2014), pp1913-1920.

CHAPTER 18

153 Ackermann, W. et al. The Influence of Glyphosate on the Microbiota and Production of Botulinum Neurotoxin During Ruminal Fermentation. *Curr Microbiol* vol. 70 (2015), pp 374.

154 Kruger, M. et al. Glyphosate suppresses the antagonistic effect of Enterococcus spp. on Clostridium botulinum. *Anaerobe*, vol. 20 (2013), pp 74-8.

155 Benbrook, C. Trends in glyphosate herbicide use in the United States and globally. Environmental Sciences Europe (2016, 28:28)

156 https://www.soilassociation.org/our-campaigns/not-in-our-bread/

157 http://www.hortweek.com/london-council-bans-contractor-use-glyphosate-parks/parks-and-gardens/article/1398373

158 Suez, J. et al. Artificial sweeteners induce glucose intolerance by altering the gut microbiota. *Nature*, vol. 514 (7521) (2014), pp181-6

159 Pérez-Cobas, A, E. et al. Gut microbiota disturbance during antibiotic therapy: a multi-omic approach. *Gut*, vol.62 (11)

160 Chassaing, B. et al. Dietary emulsifiers directly alter human microbiota composition and gene expression ex vivo potentiating intestinal inflammation. *Gut* (2017)

161 Chassaing, B. et al. Dietary emulsifiers impact the mouse gut microbiota promoting colitis and metabolic syndrome. *Nature,* vol. 519 (2015), pp92-96

CHAPTER 19

162 Zhang, Q. et al. Effect of probiotics on body weight and body-mass index: a systematic review and meta-analysis of randomized, controlled trials. *International Journal of Food Sciences and Nutrition*, vol. 67(5) (2016), pp 571

163 Ridaura, V. et al. Gut Microbiota from Twins Discordant for Obesity Modulate Metabolism in Mice. *Science*, vol. 341(6150) (2013)

164 Blaser, M. Antibiotic overuse: Stop the killing of beneficial bacteria. Nature, vol. 476, pp 393–394

CHAPTER 21

165 Stanton. C, et al. Probiotic Cheese. *International Dairy Journal*, vol. 8 (5-6) (1998), pp 491-496.

166 (WO/2002/018542) New Strains of Lactobacillus paracasei. *World Intellectual Property Organization*

167 Reynolds, J. 'Risk averse' EU industry shunning fermented food trend. Nutraingredients.com (27th February 2017)

CHAPTER 22

168 CZERUCKA, D. et al. Review article: yeast as probiotics –Saccharomyces boulardii. *Alimentary Pharmacology & Therapeutics*, vol. 26 (2007), pp 767–778.

169 Cooper, P. et al. Early Benefits of a Starter Formula Enriched in Prebiotics and Probiotics on the Gut Microbiota of Healthy Infants Born to HIV+ Mothers: A Randomized Double-Blind Controlled Trial. Clin Med Specifically to heal leaky gut:

Index